to be a nurse

D1216269

Second Edition

Evelyn Adam, R.N., M.N.
Professor Emeritus
Faculty of Nursing
University of Montreal

Appendix (Assessment Tool) by Jacinthe Pepin, R.N., M.Sc.

1991
W.B. SAUNDERS COMPANY CANADA LTD.

Philadelphia   London   Toronto   Montreal   Sydney   Tokyo

W.B. Saunders

W.B. Saunders Company Canada Limited
55 Horner Avenue
Toronto, Ontario
M8Z 4X6

W.B. Saunders
The Curtis Centre
Independence Square West
Philadelphia, PA 19106

TO BE A NURSE/2nd EDITION   ISBN 0-920513-06-9

Canadian Cataloguing in Publication Data

Adam, Evelyn
  To be a nurse

2nd ed.
Includes bibliographical references.
ISBN 0-920513-06-9

1. Nursing—Philosophy. I. Title.

RT84.5.A23 1991   610.73'01   C91-093979-6

Cover design/illustration: Glyphics/Blair Kerrigan, Heather Collins
Desktop publishing: Softprobe Computing Services Inc.
Production coordination: Francine Geraci
Printed in Canada at Hignell Printing
1 2 3 4 5   95 94 93 92 91

W.B. Saunders Company:

  55 Horner Avenue
  Toronto, Ontario M8Z 4X6, Canada

  The Curtis Centre
  Independence Square West
  Philadelphia, PA 19106, U.S.A.

  24-28 Oval Road
  London NW17DX, England

  30-52 Smidmore Street
  Marrickville, N.S.W. 2204, Australia

"Conception, my boy, *fundamental brainwork*, is what makes the difference in all art."

Rossetti, in a letter to Hall Caine.

contents

preface

There is little question that the subject of this book is of universal concern. A number of people have written and spoken along the theme, "Health is everybody's business". Parents "nurse" their children, and the children, in many cases when they grow up, "nurse" their parents when they can no longer lead independent lives.

Nursing as a voluntary or paid service has a long history. Nursing as a profession is often said to date from the middle of the nineteenth century, when Florence Nightingale demonstrated the ability of the educated nurse to affect radically the death rate of the sick and wounded British soldier in the military hospitals of the Crimea. She was, many believe, a genius.

In the provision of health care during the latter half of the twentieth century there has been a world-wide effort to define the legal boundaries of practice by doctors, dentists, nurses, social workers, and other health care providers by various names. In none of these categories has the search for a clear and useful definition been more earnest and productive of statements, differing in substance and clarity, than in nursing.

In this volume, Evelyn Adam emphasizes the flexibility of the concept of nursing underlying the small volume *Basic Principles of Nursing Care*, written by me for the International Council of Nurses in 1966; a small volume, *The Nature of Nursing*, also published in 1966; and the sixth edition of *Principles and Practice of Nursing*, published in 1978.

Evelyn Adam is explicit in describing how this concept affects practice, research, and education. Those who see its value as she does will be grateful to her for sharing exactly how it affects nursing—and other aspects of health care—wherever this concept is accepted as a reliable guide.

If health is, indeed, "everybody's business", all of us should practise self-help in an effort to achieve optimum health for ourselves, but also to make good health possible for all citizens, even as, in most countries, we make it possible for all citizens to be educated. Few now doubt the essential role of nurses in achieving what Annie W. Goodrich called "a healthy citizenry".

Virginia Henderson

foreword

Since the publication of *To Be a Nurse* (1980), my discussions with graduate students and colleagues in a variety of settings have only served to strengthen my conviction that nursing's conceptual base must be made explicit. Although our historical, religious and military roots are openly acknowledged, our conceptual frame of reference, on the contrary, has been all too often borrowed, albeit sometimes unwittingly, or discreetly allowed to sink into obscurity.

I am indebted to the many nurses who have stimulated me to keep alive the interest that was first awakened in 1969 when I had the privilege of being one of Dorothy E. Johnson's students. That remarkable professor's enthusiasm for clarifying nursing's social mandate is still felt as a profound and positive influence.

Before the term "conceptual model" became popular in nursing, Virginia Henderson's writings had already included all the elements of that structural representation. Her ideas of client wholeness and independence have lost none of their relevance for a profession that prides itself on offering an interpersonal service significant to society's health. It is therefore to Virginia Henderson that I owe the inspiration for both editions of this book. They have been written in the hope of increasing nurses' awareness of the far-reaching influence of their way of conceptualizing our professional discipline.

Evelyn Adam
Professor Emeritus
Faculty of Nursing
University of Montreal

introduction

The nursing profession has existed, according to the writers of its history, since the time of the caveman, who, returning wounded from the hunt, had his sores dressed by the cavewoman. Closer to our own era, "modern nursing" is said to have begun with Florence Nightingale and the opening of her first school in 1860 (Dolan, 1978; Bullough & Bullough, 1971). Nurse historians also underline the development of nursing in Canada from the very beginning of the French colony and emphasize the work of Jeanne Mance, who began her nursing career in Canada with the founding of Montreal in 1642. American nursing history is also well documented.

Despite our long history, our social mission today is far from clear. For some, within the profession as well as outside it, the nurse is the physician's helper—more poetically described as the "handmaiden of the physician." For others, the nurse is an autonomous professional who also carries out medical orders. Between these two extremes the role of the nurse is perceived and described in many different ways; the nurse herself,* until recently, has seen little necessity to justify her reason for being.

However, nurses and their role have been the subject of several sociological studies. Mauksch (1966) compares the nursing profession to a sheet of rolled-out dough from which many cookies have been cut; these cut-out cookies are rising and browning independently in the oven and represent the traditional functions of the nurse that have been taken over by new groups of health workers. What is left of the sheet of dough constitutes nursing.

The role of the nurse is of course constantly evolving. If the change is influenced on the one hand by the appearances of new groups of specialists, it is on the other hand due to the deliberate

---

* For convenience sake, the feminine is used in reference to the nurse. Both men and women are members of the nursing profession.

reaching out by nurses for new and less traditional functions. There has been a tendency among nurses in the last several years to seek legal authorization to perform certain acts that, traditionally and officially, have been regarded as the prerogative of the physician. As nurses acquire jurisdiction of these tasks, the accompanying tendency is for them to abandon some of their own traditional tasks to nursing assistants or health care aides.

Returning to the analogy of the cookie dough, we are confronted with the evidence that many cookies have been cut out, much of the remaining dough has been "given" to others, and the legal battle for the new and sought-after dough has not been completely won. Looked at in this way, nursing does not present a pretty picture. The situation does, however, provide us with an excellent opportunity to ask ourselves, individually and collectively, some very basic questions: "Who am I? What am I trying to achieve? What is it exactly that I do?"

This writer believes that nursing is a worthwhile service and one that is generally considered important by most societies; while recognizing that nurses collaborate in the carrying out of doctors' orders and with other health professionals in various ways, the writer also believes that nurses have, as well, an independent social mission to accomplish.

It is highly probable that nurses will continue for some time to come to carry out various tasks asked of them by physicians for the last century and more; at least *that* part of nursing is abundantly clear. However, the *independent* part of nursing is, on the contrary, not nearly as clear either for the general public or for nurses themselves. The oft-heard "nursing is an art and a science" is not easily defended; it is difficult to describe exactly what constitutes the "science" of nursing, and the "art" is frequently explained by a series of well-defined tasks, many of which, no matter how independent the nurse's performance, are nonetheless the application of medical knowledge. Yet nurses in general, from the most radical to the most conservative, usually agree that nursing is not just carrying out doctors' orders; nursing is "more than that." It is the "more than that" that is crying out for clarification.

The purpose of this book is to attempt to answer that cry for clarity. Written for students and graduates in any setting, this book will describe the necessary elements of a complete and explicit way of looking at nursing, present the writings of Virginia Henderson as a conceptual model, and discuss the implications of such a theoretical framework in relation to the three general fields of nursing activity: practice, education, and research. Each field has an important component of administration.

chapter 1

a frame of reference for nursing

It has become almost trite to say that the world about us is rapidly and constantly changing and therefore requires of everyone considerable powers of adaptation. What was sufficient for our needs a few centuries ago no longer satisfies us today and what was very suitable even a few years ago is no longer acceptable by current standards.

The nursing profession, seemingly a necessary part of many societies for hundreds of years, is no exception to the evolutionary process. If the nurse of bygone years was relatively content to have her identity merged inseparably with that of other health professionals, today's nurse is striving for recognition as a professional in her own right. The growing complexity of modern health services obliges the nurse to make more explicit her specific contribution, as a member of the interdisciplinary team, to the health of the community. Her efforts at clarifying her role are as necessary for her personal satisfaction as they are for explaining the nature of her professional service to a demanding public.

All health workers have of course a common goal: the preservation and improvement of the client or beneficiary's health and well-being. This very broad goal encompasses the more specific goal of each of the health disciplines. The members of each discipline make known their particular professional goal, thus justifying their presence on the health team. By both their words and their deeds they make clear their specific contribution to the improvement of the population's health.

That the nurse, as a full-fledged member of the team, should explain the nature of her particular service to society does not mean that she will refuse henceforth to share certain functions with other health professionals or cease to accept certain delegated activities. On the contrary, making very clear her own special contribution can only clarify that part of her contribution that she shares with others; defining the parameters of her own profession can only underline the independence of her colleagues. The interdependence that is so highly valued between health workers can be realized only if a minimum of independence has been achieved by each of the professions involved.

A frame of reference, such as described in the following chapter, allows the members of the nursing profession to state precisely the nature of their contribution to the large and complex arena of health services. Such a conceptual framework offers direction for nursing practice, education, and research, including the administrative component of each. The framework is therefore useful, if not essential, to every nurse, not only in her professional role as a member of the health team, but also in her role as an individual person. As a health professional she can clearly explain to her co-workers and to the general public the nature of her service to society. If the nurse needs to convince various authorities that she must be included in newly formed health oriented groups, she will refer to the same frame of reference to justify her insistence.

As an individual member of society, the nurse also finds her conceptual framework helpful. The nurse of today is no longer the same member of society that she once was. No longer content to play a subordinate role either as a woman (and the majority of nurses are women) or as a nurse, she now claims equal status with other health professionals. Dissatisfied with the salary of another era, she is now requesting, often helped by her collective bargaining unit, a salary commensurate with her responsibilities. Such modern demands, legitimate as they may be, are accompanied by the serious obligation of knowing what the nurse's part in societal health really is and the equally serious responsibility of explaining it.

While it is true that most nurses really wish to offer valuable help to mankind, their professional commitment is sometimes openly questioned; nurses have been accused of indifference, unkindness, or worse still, of downright negligence. Becker (1969) discusses the concept of commitment:

> ... a person is committed when we observe him pursuing a consistent line of activity in a sequence of varied situations. Consistent activity persists over time. Further, even though the actor may engage in a variety of disparate acts, he sees them as essentially consistent; from his point of view they serve him in pursuit of the same goal. (p. 264)

A specific conceptual framework would contribute to a nurse's commitment by providing a single unifying goal to which the nurse can relate, and would thus contribute to the nurse's personal satisfaction as well as that of the public she wishes to serve.

Every nurse has, of course, a personal frame of reference or her own private concept of nursing. It seems quite impossible *not* to have an idea of what it means to be a nurse. It is often true, however, that the nurse cannot easily put into words the mental image of nursing that she carries in her head, for that picture is not clear enough to be expressed in words. A blurred picture needs to be clearly focused; a precise frame of reference does exactly that—focuses the picture so that it is cleanly outlined and gives a complete and explicit conceptualization.

It is still of interest today to reread the description of nursing's mission written by Florence Nightingale (1859) over one hundred years ago:

> It is often thought that medicine is the curative process. It is no such thing; medicine is the surgery of functions, as surgery proper is that of limbs and organs. Neither can do anything but remove obstructions; neither can cure; nature alone cures. ... And what nursing has to do in either case, is to put the patient in the best condition for nature to act upon him. (p. 74-75)

While we still find much to admire in Miss Nightingale's vision of nursing, today we require more clarity and precision so as to put it in focus. These two qualities can be found in a number of the various conceptual frameworks that experienced nurses have made explicit. None of these conceptions of nursing is perfect—nor "right"! Each one is the work of a human being and, as such, demonstrates that perfection is not of this world. It is nonetheless true that each conception offers clarity and precision about nursing's reason for being. The nurse administrator of a curriculum, nursing service, or research project, as well as the teachers, practitioners and researchers themselves, may choose to adopt one of these conceptions.

The components of a complete and explicit conceptual framework are discussed in the next chapter.

chapter 2

the components of a conceptual model

In this chapter, the reader will find described the essential elements of a conceptual model. These are assumptions, values and major units.

The expression "conceptual model", used for some time in other disciplines (sociology, mathematics, etc.), is relatively new in the vocabulary of nurses. If the term has been recently acquired, the idea is not at all new, since every nurse has always had a personal way of conceptualizing or looking at her own profession.

The conceptual model for any discipline is a structural representation of reality and is clearly not the reality itself (Riehl & Roy, 1980). Everyone looks at the world around him through his own conceptual "glasses". For example, a person who finds himself faced with a plate of fresh oysters may regard them with great relish, while the person seated beside him may react with horror at the prospect of having to swallow *that* reality.

People may have very different conceptions of a given discipline, much as they may differ radically in their conceptions of success, happiness, marriage, or even of what constitutes an appropriate car. Some people may "see" nursing as medical assistance; others may have a mental image of nursing as an autonomous profession.

A conceptual model *for* any discipline is a conception *of* that discipline, but one that is clear and precise enough to offer direction for its practice, research and education. Not all conceptions of a discipline are explicit enough to warrant the appellation "conceptual model". When a conception of a discipline is so blurred that it cannot be put into words, it is not a conceptual model.

When the word "model" is not qualified by "conceptual", it may mean many things: a good example (a model student), a method of management (business model), a physical model (a plastic model of the heart, an airplane model), or a fashion model.

While a conceptual model may be correctly referred to as a conceptual framework or frame of reference, the inverse is not necessarily true. Some frames of reference and frameworks may be philosophies or theories (Adam, 1985). A conceptual model for a discipline is useful only to that discipline, whereas philosophies and theories are useful to various different disciplines.

A conceptual model is not a definition of the discipline; it is a conception of what the discipline could be or should be.

A conception of a discipline is said to be "complete" when it contains all the essential elements of a model and "explicit" when those elements are formally and distinctly stated.

According to Johnson (see Riehl & Roy, 1980), the elements of a conceptual model are:

1. the assumptions
2. the beliefs and values
3. the major units:
   a. the ideal and limited goal of the profession
   b. the beneficiary of the professional service
   c. the social role of the professional
   d. the source of difficulty of the beneficiary
   e. the intervention of the professional
   f. the consequences

We shall now look at these elements in detail:

1. the assumptions

The *assumptions* make up the theoretical and scientific basis of the conceptual model. The assumptions chosen for the theoretical foundation of the model may come from a particular theory or practice or both. They have either been verified in the development of the theory or are at least amenable to verification. The assumptions are the suppositions that are taken for granted by those who wish to use the model; they are the "how" of the model, its foundation.*

2. the beliefs and values

The *beliefs and values* constitute the "why" of the model and are not subject to the criteria of truth. They must, however, reflect the value system of the larger society that the profession wishes to serve. The beliefs and values inherent in a particular model must be shared by the members of the profession who wish to adopt the model; if these cannot be accepted, the members of that profession must choose another conceptual model whose underlying value system would be more compatible with their own.**

3. the major units

The *major units* are the "what" of the conceptual model. They are the life of the model and animate the professional activities of those who see the profession in the same way. The major units of a model for nursing offer a clear conception of nursing in any setting and at any time. They give meaning to the various actions carried out by the members of the profession. Specifically, these major units comprise the following:

---

* As a very simple example, this writer asks the reader to recognize and accept the following assumptions:
  1. every nurse is capable of conceptualizing
  2. her personal conception of nursing is often unclear and incomplete. These assumptions do not come from a particular theory; they are, however, amenable to verification by having nurses pass the appropriate tests and they are the premises on which this book is written.

** To continue the simple example, this writer believes that nurses play an important role in society and that their role warrants clarification. This belief represents the "why" of this volume and the reader who does not share the belief may be tempted to read no further.

a. *The goal of the profession* is the end to which the members of the profession strive. The goal is ideal and at the same time limited. It is "ideal" because it represents the ideal that all members of the profession would like to achieve and "limited" because it delineates the parameters of the profession. The members strive toward an ideal, even though they do not always succeed in attaining it. At the same time, since they cannot be all things to all people, they realistically recognize the limitations of their service. While the goal of nursing is a specific one, it must nonetheless be congruent with the common goal of all members of the health team. The specific goal of nursing justifies the presence of the nurse among the other health professionals. The nurse pursues her ideal goal in her professional activities at all times but since her ideal goal is defined as to scope, she does not attempt to do everything.

b. *The target of action* is the object of the profession's activity. For helping or service professions, the target of action is the person or group of persons towards whom the professional directs his attention. That person or group of persons (the potential or actual *client(s)* of the professional service) is conceptualized in a certain way by the professional and that mental picture is the second major unit of the model. The nurse must have a clear mental image of her client, whether he is well or ill. If another member of the health team sees the client mainly as a biophysiological system with the subsystems being cardiovascular, gastrointestinal, and so forth, does the nurse also see the client that way or does she see him according to her own particular frame of reference?

c. *The social role of the professional* is the role in society played by the members of the discipline in question. The role must necessarily be recognized and accepted by the larger society, for if it were otherwise, the service would probably disappear, since helping professions usually exist in response to needs of the society.

The public requests the services of a lawyer because that professional can skilfully play the role of defender of rights; the same public consults a physician because he is seen as playing a curative or healing role. In a conceptual model for nursing, this third major unit makes explicit the social role of the nurse.

d. *The source of difficulty* refers to the probable origin of the client's difficulty; one with which the professional, because of his education and experience, is prepared to cope. This fourth unit points out, in abstract terms, the profession's jurisdiction. The many problems that a client of a health care system may have cannot all be solved by one health worker; each professional has a particular sphere of competence. The probable origin of those client problems which the nurse is prepared to solve must be made explicit.

e. *The intervention* is further divided into:

1. The *focus or centre of the intervention*, *i.e.*, the focus of the professional's attention at the moment he intervenes with a client. The patient or beneficiary is perceived as an extremely complex individual; within that complexity only one aspect can receive all the professional's attention at any given moment. Even though the whole person is not forgotten, the particular action of the moment must be directed toward a part of the whole, since no one person can do everything at the same time. As a concrete example, a dentist who considers his client as a complex whole may concentrate his attention at a given moment on the enamel of one tooth, while at another moment he might direct his attention to the dental health behaviour of the same client.

2. The *modes of intervention* are the means the professional has at his disposal. Actions themselves are not suggested. The *mode* of intervention is suggested and indicates in

abstract terms the form that subsequent concrete actions may take. For example, medicine's intervention modes are surgical, radiological, etc. A conceptual model for nursing indicates the means that are available to the nurse when she wishes to intervene.

f. *The consequences* are the desired results of the professional activities and must be congruent with the ideal goal. Some professions are able to predict undesirable consequences as well. The latter are those consequences which may be produced as unwanted side effects even as the desired consequences are obtained.

Such a detailed conceptual framework (assumptions, values and major units) can be easily and clearly communicated and therefore compared with other ways of looking at reality both within the same profession and among professions. The words used are, of course, abstract terms, for the mental picture *is* an abstraction. For the helping professions, conception reaches the real world in the orientation it suggests for practice, education, and research within that particular profession. Abstract terms provide the guidelines for concrete action and these guidelines, whose cohesiveness and inner logic are thus assured, give direction to the practitioner, educator, and researcher.

Several experienced nurses have made known their mental picture of nursing. These various conceptions differ from one another in their assumptions although they resemble one another in their beliefs and sometimes in some of the major units.

The day will perhaps come when one conceptual model for nursing will be unanimously accepted by nurses around the world. At present we are far from such consensus; the way nurses see their profession seems to vary considerably from one school of nursing to another and from one health establishment to another. Indeed, for the moment, such a variety of mental pictures is preferable in order to judge, one day, which is the most socially significant, congruent, and useful.

Much less acceptable, however, is the situation where *within one* school or health agency the way of conceptualizing nursing varies from nurse to nurse or remains non-communicable because, as a group of nurses, they have not adopted a complete and explicit frame of reference to guide their activities. Since they do not have a clear and precise idea of nursing, not only do they have difficulty communicating with each other, but they have trouble explaining to the public, students, and other health professionals the nature of nursing's contribution to the health of the community.

The purpose of this book is to present one complete and explicit conception of the service that nurses offer to society. The following chapter describes one way of conceptualizing nursing, drawn from the writings of Virginia Henderson.

chapter 3

one way of looking at nursing

Virginia Henderson, an internationally known American nurse, has long exerted a powerful influence on the profession. Her concept of nursing is presented here as a conceptual model, that is, a frame of reference made up of assumptions, values, and major units.

assumptions

The assumptions that form the theoretical foundation of Virginia Henderson's vision of nursing are drawn in part from the works of Thorndike (1940), an American psychologist, and in part from Miss Henderson's experience in rehabilitation. There are three assumptions (Henderson, 1964, 1966):

1. Every individual strives for and desires independence.
2. Every individual is a complex whole, made up of fundamental needs.
3. When a need is not satisfied, the individual is not complete, whole, or independent.

The word "need" calls for a definition. In the context of Henderson's writings, a need is a *requirement*, rather than a *lack*.* In the present volume, the word need is used in that positive sense—a necessity or a requirement.

values

The beliefs underlying Virginia Henderson's conception of nursing are also three in number (Henderson, 1966):

1. The nurse has a unique function, although she shares certain functions with other professionals.

---

* Letter from V. Henderson, June, 1977.

2. When the nurse takes over the physician's role, she delegates her primary function to inadequately prepared personnel. The nurse may be tempted to assume the physician's role but when she gives in to the temptation she delegates her own role to personnel less prepared than herself.

3. Society wants and expects this service (nursing) from the nurse and no other worker is as able, or willing, to give it.

major units

The major units of Henderson's model (Henderson, 1966) are:

1. **The goal of nursing** is to maintain or to restore the client's independence in the satisfaction of his fundamental needs.* This goal, congruent with the goal common to the entire health team, makes clear the nurse's specific contribution to the preservation and improvement of health.

2. **The client** of the nurse's services is a complex whole, an entity presenting fourteen fundamental needs.

The needs that are common to all human beings, well or sick, are the following (not in order of importance):

1. Breathe normally.
2. Eat and drink adequately.
3. Eliminate body wastes.
4. Move and maintain desirable postures.
5. Sleep and rest.
6. Select suitable clothes—dress and undress.
7. Maintain body temperature within normal range by adjusting clothing and modifying the environment.
8. Keep the body clean and well groomed and protect the integument.
9. Avoid dangers in the environment and avoid injuring others.

---

* For convenience sake, the masculine is used in reference to the client. "Client" includes the well person and the sick patient.

10. Communicate with others in expressing emotions, needs, fears, or opinions.

11. Worship according to one's faith.

12. Work in such a way that there is a sense of accomplishment.

13. Play or participate in various forms of recreation.

14. Learn, discover, or satisfy the curiosity that leads to normal development and health and use the available health facilities.

While the fourteen needs are common to all clients, individual differences in the specific needs which derive from them vary greatly from one person to another. The complex "whole" is therefore much more than the sum of fourteen basic needs; the "holistic" vision of the client allows for countless needs, each of which is in itself complex. The "wholeness" of the client is contingent on the satisfaction of his needs and the nurse's goal is his independence in need satisfaction.

3. **The role of the nurse** is a complementary-supplementary one. This role consists of "substituting for what the patient lacks to make him complete, whole, independent." (Henderson, 1968, p. 4) The nurse "is temporarily the consciousness of the unconscious, the love of life for the suicidal, the leg of the amputee, the eyes of the newly blind, a means of locomotion for the infant, knowledge and confidence for the young mother, a 'mouthpiece' for those too weak or withdrawn to speak, and so on." (p. 4)

4. **The source of difficulty**, or the probable origin of those problems known as nursing problems, is either a lack of knowledge, will or strength.

5. **The intervention:** The focus, or centre of attention, of the nurse's action is the client's deficit or area of dependence. A need that the client cannot himself satisfy calls for an intervention by the nurse who, concentrating her attention on complementing and supplementing strength, will, and knowledge, attempts to satisfy the need in order to maintain the client's wholeness.

For example, if a young mother cannot alone satisfy her need to care for her first-born (fundamental need to work in such a way as to have a sense of accomplishment) because she lacks some of the necessary knowledge, the nurse concentrates on that area of dependence and attempts to complete the young mother's knowledge so that she will become independent in that regard.

The modes of intervention available to the nurse are: replace, complete, substitute, add, reinforce, increase. The concrete action that derives from these abstract terms is the intervention itself.

6. **The desired consequences**, in the short term, are satisfaction of the client's needs; in the middle or long term, they are increased independence in need satisfaction and, in some cases, a peaceful death.

the fourteen basic needs

The preceding assumptions, values and major units make up a complete and explicit way of looking at nursing, whether the nurse is working with well or sick people, with children or adults, in the delivery room or in the coronary care unit, in the home or in the hospital. The variables in each situation are of course very different, depending on whether the beneficiary of the nursing service is a school-child or a factory worker, a patient hospitalized because of a fracture or because of a mental illness; in all cases, however, the service offered by the nurse is that of maintaining or restoring the client's independence in the satisfaction of his fourteen fundamental needs.

A cursory examination of the fourteen fundamental needs reveals that those which, at first glance, seem to be especially influenced by human biology (age, sex, genetic makeup) and physiology (functioning of organs) also have important psycho-socio-cultural dimensions (including political and economic factors). The inverse is also true. Needs which seem to belong to a psycho-social category have, as well, bio-physiological components.

The cornerstone of nursing's social mission, according to Henderson's way of looking at the profession, is to foster independence in the satisfaction of fourteen basic human needs. A brief discussion of each of the fourteen needs follows:*

1. Breathe normally

The bio-physiological aspect of this "necessity" is obvious in the cellular and pulmonary exchange and in the intimate relationship between the respiratory apparatus and the circulatory, neurological and muscular networks. The psycho-socio-cultural component is important. Emotions such as fear, anger and grief influence respiratory rate and depth. Feelings of pleasure may accompany breathing freely of clean air or of agreeable odours. Those who practise transcendental meditation and yoga attach a special importance to breathing. Smoking, still popular today, and sometimes publicized as adding to a person's sexual attractiveness, was not always a respectable habit in some cultures and is once more frowned upon, or frankly rejected, by certain groups.

Independence in the satisfaction of the need to breathe is therefore something individual and personal. The special needs of a newborn are different from those of an adult; similarly, the breathing requirements of an athlete are not those of a post-operative patient in intensive care. The need to breathe is closely related to all the other fundamental needs; for some it is particularly linked to the need to avoid danger (the industrial worker) and for others it is specifically connected to the need to express emotions (anxiety crisis).

2. Eat and drink adequately

Independence in the satisfaction of the need for food and liquids is evidently complex. The bio-physiological aspect includes using the hand to transport appropriate nourishment to the mouth, chewing and swallowing, digestion and absorption, as well as caloric or special requirements, as in the case of a person with diabetes or anemia.

---

* For a more exhaustive study, the reader is encouraged to consult Henderson and Nite (1978).

Psycho-socio-cultural dimensions are numerous: racial preferences, religious or national habits as reflected by different meal times and choice of food, the meaning that individuals may attach to food (love, comfort, punishment), and popular attitudes about breast feeding, food fads, and current fashion in clothes.

As with all of the fourteen requirements, the need for nourishment is linked to various other needs, such as the need to communicate, eliminate wastes and accomplish something useful. It also varies with the degree of maturity of the individual.

3. Eliminate body wastes

This need includes elimination by kidneys, intestines, lungs and skin. In some situations, artificial orifices (*e.g.*, tracheostomy, colostomy) are special ways of ridding the body of wastes.

The bio-physiological component is mechanical, chemical, hormonal and nervous and differs greatly with age and state of health. Psycho-socio-cultural aspects are equally varied. Emotions, both pleasant and unpleasant, influence perspiration and CO_2 elimination, urinary frequency and the quality and quantity of stools. Socio-cultural heritage has its impact on the requirements of privacy for eliminating, the meaning attached to excreta, the attitudes of parents toward toilet training and the association both children and adults make between the sexual and eliminative organs.

While the basic need to eliminate is common to all humans, the individual variations are multiple and as with other needs, independence relative to this need satisfaction serves to underline individual differences.

4. Move and maintain desirable postures

From a bio-physiological point of view, it is clear that independence in satisfying this need differs from the small child to the adult and that independence for a paraplegic paralysed for ten years is very different from that of an Olympic runner. Freedom of movement and freedom to assume or avoid certain postures are directly related to such subsystems as the musculo-skeletal, cardio-vascular, nervous, and so forth.

As for the psycho-socio-cultural variables, differences may be considerable. Emotional health or state of mind is reflected, consciously or unconsciously, in body posture and movement; body language, as an expression of the psychic vitality of the person, is a constant reminder of the union of soma and psyche. Social customs and cultural patterns determine, in large part, the relative importance given to "military academy" posture for young men, to the way a "well-brought-up" young lady sits and walks, and to "acceptable" body movements in the House of Commons or at a discotheque, to give only a few examples.

Satisfaction of this need means multiple and complex activities and is closely linked to the satisfaction of other needs such as doing useful work and seeking recreation. Health problems render the individuality of motor activity even more complex; for example, walking on crutches, shifting position every hour, or elevating lower limbs when in a sitting position.

5. Sleep and rest

The biological and physiological aspects of this human need vary with age and conditions of health. A small child, for example, needs more sleep than an adolescent, and a man recovering from a myocardial infarction has different rest requirements from his neighbour who has suffered a broken leg in a car accident. The quality of sleep, and of physical and mental rest, is closely related to cardio-respiratory, gastro-intestinal and neuro-muscular functioning. A person deprived of sleep, or even deprived of dreaming, may develop physical and emotional problems.

Regarding the psycho-socio-cultural dimension, sleep and rest are affected by emotions and social "obligations." For example, contrast the behaviours of certain sub-groups who use drugs to remain awake or to fall asleep to those who practise yoga and transcendental meditation to regulate their sleep and relaxation functions naturally.

To be independent in satisfying the need for rest and sleep does not have the same significance for everyone, nor even for one person at all times. For example, a young woman who ordinarily sleeps six hours a night may find she requires much more sleep in the early months of pregnancy.

6. Select suitable clothes—dress and undress

This human need has many different forms for well people as well as for those who are ill. From a bio-physiological point of view, daily activities in dressing and undressing require considerable neuromuscular ability and also exemplify the differences between young and old. Health problems may create very personal needs, *e.g.*, following a mastectomy, a woman is preoccupied by the prosthesis and by her underclothing, while a hemiplegic is concerned with finding clothing that can be put on and taken off with one hand.

Psycho-socio-cultural aspects are almost without limit. The choice of a certain way of dressing becomes a means of asserting one's personality and sexuality. Religious and cultural groups often have specific dress requirements (*e.g.*, veil, turban, caftan), current fashion has made "jeans" known around the world, and socio-cultural mores often dictate the state of dress, or undress, at the beach.

The psycho-social component of this need demands special attention from the nurse when a client is undergoing diagnostic tests or receiving treatment. Respecting the patient's modesty, according to his age, sex and socio-cultural group, requires using screens, curtains and drapes or towels. Ignoring this aspect of care means that a fundamental human need is not satisfied.

7. Maintain body temperature within normal range

Maintaining a normal temperature is largely bio-physiological; age is an important factor, as is individual tolerance to environmental changes. Body temperature is affected by exercise, the type of clothing worn, circulation and nutrition, hypothalamic control and biological rhythms (circadian, lunar, etc.).

Since emotions also affect body temperature, the psychology of the individual is an important variable. Anxiety can increase a person's temperature and is closely associated with the socio-cultural position of the individual.

8. Keep the body clean and well groomed and protect the integument

Independence in personal hygiene is obviously contingent on the physical capacity to perform a number of fine movements as well as on the biological factors of age and sex. Individual requirements vary for the youngster at puberty, the aging person, the menstruating girl, and the uncircumcised boy.

Mental and emotional health are reflected in the condition of the skin and hair and in the attention the individual gives to his grooming. Feelings of well-being are increased when personal needs for cleanliness and grooming are satisfied. Emotions affect perspiration and the production of certain secretions. Standards of cleanliness vary from one society to another and within a culture from one time period to another. The influence of psycho-socio-cultural factors on toilet training is an important example.

With an alteration in a person's health new cleanliness needs may appear, *e.g.*, the requirements of someone who has just had a colostomy are not those of someone with an infectious skin disease; the diabetic child learns special care for his feet; the hemiplegic patiently learns how to wash his un-paralysed arm.

9. Avoid dangers in the environment and avoid injuring others

Avoiding danger from both the external and internal environment in order to assure physical and psychological security is also a fundamental human need of great complexity.

Bio-physiologically, independence may require avoiding a particular food, medication, or physical activity; *e.g.*, one child must follow a gluten-free diet while another must carefully avoid any contact with pollen. For a hospitalized patient, avoiding danger may be as simple as raising the bed rails or as complicated as isolation with reversed technique; in some cases it may mean protecting the patient who has suicidal tendencies.

For the well person as for the ill, the satisfaction of this need has important psycho-social connotations. Providing psychological security may take the form of a telephone call or the continuous presence, for a time, of a close relative. Social isolation or cultural alienation may be neutralized by such diverse means as listening to rock music, conversing with someone who speaks the same native tongue or who comes from the same cultural group, or having a particular cultural custom or object respected by others.

Avoiding danger, or preventing accidents of all kinds, is inseparable from each of the other thirteen fundamental needs and, as such, is a highly personal and individual necessity for all human beings.

10. **Communicate with others in expressing emotions, needs, fears, or opinions**

This basic human need has long attracted the attention of many professional groups. Every year new books are written about the various aspects of human communication and interpersonal relationships.

Communication has biological aspects. Verbal or non-verbal expression of one's sexual characteristics through posture, clothing or movements is an example. Communication is physiological in that verbal communication includes articulating (lips and tongue) and making sounds (larynx). Non-verbal expression includes the physical ability to gesture, change facial expression, and adopt a variety of postures.

The psycho-socio-cultural dimension is evident in the content which a person chooses to communicate or not communicate: feelings, opinions, hopes, dreams, etc. It is socially "acceptable" or culturally "allowed" to express certain emotions or to express them in a given way and that acceptability determines, at least to some extent, how an individual expresses outwardly his inner self. While some cartoonists underline the reserve and euphemisms of anglo-saxons, others point out the emotionalism and hyperbole of latins.

Communication includes the sexuality of the individual. Considered in a broad sense, this important dimension of a human being is revealed from infancy to very old age: self-assertion, personality, choice of clothing, social relationships, etc. Viewed in the more restricted sense of genital activity, human sexuality constitutes a privileged form of verbal and non-verbal communication.

In good health or in sickness, young and old have a multitude of things to communicate to others. When a client cannot, for various reasons, satisfy the need himself, the nurse must help him to express what he wishes to express and help him find new ways of communicating when formerly used modes are no longer possible. This can be a very difficult task and it underscores the importance of careful professional preparation.

11. Worship according to one's faith

The need to practise one's religion includes the practice of any ideology or spirituality important to a person, even though that ideology may be considered a-religious.

The bio-physiological element is seen in the various gestures, postures, or movements necessary to worship. Penance may require the person to kneel or to fast; some religions have their men circumcised, others forbid particular foods, and still others refuse certain forms of medical treatment.

Religious practices follow, to some extent, psycho-social changes and inter-cultural attitudes; churches become more democratic or less so, inter-racial and cross-cultural marriages are forbidden or permitted, the obligation to attend Sunday mass may be fulfilled on Saturday, and so forth.

An alteration in health may bring about an increase or decrease in an individual's religious practice. Whatever the age of the patient, the respect of this fundamental need, as indeed for all needs, requires that nurses receive a liberal education and develop their skills in empathic interpersonal relations.

12. Work in such a way that there is a sense of accomplishment

At all stages of life, people have a basic need to accomplish something useful. Learning to walk, studying and working are only three examples. Some accomplishments are sex-linked (biology), but most are rather associated with physiological ability and psycho-social development. Cultural norms affect the satisfaction of this need. For example, ambitious individuals in a highly industrialized society may require, to satisfy their need for accomplishment, something quite different from individuals of another culture who value artistic or philosophical expression above all other things.

To be independent in the satisfaction of this important need varies from the composer to the politician and from the mother to the fashion model. Often the same person can accomplish useful work in more than one area. Health problems may permanently or temporarily keep an individual from the activities that provide him with a sense of accomplishment. Satisfaction in this area is closely related to other needs such as learning, communicating, and moving about.

13. Play or participate in various forms of recreation

Although common to all human beings, the need for play and diversion is satisfied in very different ways from childhood to old age and from one adult to another. Independence in recreation has bio-physiological elements, *e.g.*, a person born blind finds different forms of play than people with eyesight, and physiological status may decide an individual's choice between reading and downhill skiing.

Recreational satisfaction is strongly influenced by such socio-cultural phenomena as television and the leisure society. In addition, emotions may determine the choice of how leisure time is spent and the recreation chosen influences, in its turn, the emotional status of the person. Thus, an angry man may rid himself very satisfactorily of the unpleasant feeling by attacking a punching-bag, while another may find that he is experiencing less anxiety after a game of baseball with his children.

The need for play and diversion in no way disappears when a person is ill. On the contrary, periods of relaxing recreation take on a special importance and should be planned along with other aspects of care.

14. Learn, discover or satisfy curiosity

Although the need to learn and satisfy one's curiosity may be more apparent in childhood and during the years of formal education, it is basic to all humans at all stages of their life. Learning is related to intelligence (biology) and to the five senses (physiology), and these factors are of great importance in need satisfaction.

Psycho-socio-cultural factors are seen in the individual's desire to learn, his capacity to tolerate intellectual stimulation, and the value his socio-cultural group places on education. Political and economic dimensions of a social reality include day nurseries, televised messages, continuing education possibilities, and government scholarships. All have their impact on the satisfaction of the need to learn.

The health of a society may be indicative of its need to learn health habits. Any health problem that occurs, or its prevention before it occurs, can create new learning needs. One client needs to learn how to apply a dressing, another how to assert himself more effectively, and a third how to inject his own insulin and reconcile his dietary restrictions with his business luncheons. The need to learn is closely tied to the need to accomplish and the need to play; it may well be an essential condition for recovering independence in the satisfaction of any of the fourteen needs.

In summary, the fourteen basic human needs have many different ramifications according to the individual's state of health, maturity, and personal and cultural habits. Each of the fundamental needs has a biological, physiological, psychological, sociological and cultural dimension. The fourteen needs form a whole; to consider any of them to the exclusion of the others is to negate the whole, and to try to separate the physical from the psychic needs is not only a waste of time but actually harmful. When the person is seen as a whole, it becomes quite useless to discuss physical health and mental health as though the two could be separated.

Following Henderson's conceptual framework, the ideal and limited goal of nursing is the independence of the client in the satisfaction of his needs.

This chapter has presented Virginia Henderson's "concept of nursing" within the structure of a conceptual model. As with any other conception of nursing, the nurse carries it in her head, in her mind's eye; it is her mental image of her professional discipline. Speaking figuratively, the nurse's way of looking at her discipline is situated in her occipital (visual) lobe.

The abstraction that is a conceptual model is linked to reality by means of a systematic method. That systematic process is discussed in the following chapter.

chapter 4

independence nursing and the systematic process

Although the expression "nursing process" appeared in the American nursing literature during the fifties, it became prevalent only in the mid-sixties (Yura & Walsh, 1973). The term may have seemed new; its meaning was not. Without being able to name each step of the process, nurses had nonetheless always tried, more or less intuitively perhaps, to explore the parameters of a situation before deciding to take action, and then to evaluate the efficiency of their behaviour. Whether they were "private-duty" or "visiting" nurses, in the hospital or in the home, they were accustomed to collect information in order to plan the day and judge the results of their nursing care.

With the expression "nursing process" officially recognized, and its various steps clearly identified, the process could be studied, analysed, and even taught. No longer an intuitive way of proceeding, the process became known to a large number of nurses as both a practical and educational method.

The process itself, without the adjective "nursing", is of course used by many disciplines. It is even used instinctively by a great many people in the numerous decisions that must be made during the course of a single day. Many individuals collect information about the weather in order to decide what to wear for the day or whether or not to take the car to work, and a short time later they are in a position to judge the wisdom of their decision. Used in the sense of a series of actions or operations, a process is a systematic way of proceeding toward an end, a systematic method, a methodological operation, a dynamic procedure.

Henderson (1982) points out that the analytical process is no more peculiar to nursing than to medicine, social work, or physiotherapy. Henderson questions not only the title "nursing process" but also the way the method is now used and what it has come to mean.

It is of some interest, from an historical viewpoint, that in 1967 a committee involved in curriculum development identified the steps of the nursing process as perception, communication, interpretation, intervention, and evaluation. In the same year, teachers of nursing at the Catholic University of America named four steps in the nursing process: assessing, planning, implementing, evaluating (Yura & Walsh, 1973).

Today, although the terms may differ slightly depending on the writer, it is generally agreed that the "nursing" process has five sequential steps:

1. data collection
2. interpretation of data
3. planning the intervention
4. implementation
5. evaluation

The process is circular. No sooner is the fifth step completed than the first step must be undertaken again; new data require an interpretation, which leads in turn to another intervention, etc. This cyclic process comes to an end only when the client-nurse relationship is terminated.

The nursing process is applicable in any setting, in any frame of reference and within any philosophy (Yura & Walsh, 1973). Whatever conceptual model she uses, the nurse proceeds in the same systematic manner, giving equal importance to each of the five steps. A chain is only as strong as its weakest link (Aspinall, 1976).

Each link of the chain will now be studied, following the conceptual framework described in chapter 3.

data collection

Regardless of the frame of reference, the sources of information are the same:

a. the client and his family
b. the members of the health team
c. the client's file
d. reference books and manuals
e. the nurse's knowledge and experience

The most valuable source of information is the client and his family, and the most efficient ways of obtaining the desired information are direct observation and the interview.

The interview may be structured or unstructured, and conducted with or without the help of an assessment tool. The latter will be discussed later.

The important question that must be asked whenever a nurse decides to do a nursing assessment, or even thinks of collecting data from a client, is: what information must be collected? In other words, what does a nurse need to know about a patient in order to care for him? What data constitute nursing data and are not collected by another health worker, except, of course, for some inevitable overlapping?

The answer to this important question is found in the mental image the nurse has of her own profession. If that concept clearly indicates that her goal is to maintain or restore the client's independence in the satisfaction of his fourteen fundamental needs, it follows that she must seek information about his independence status relative to those fourteen areas. A mother of a large family may not, for example, be independent in her need to learn and accomplish the useful work of feeding her family on a restricted budget because she does not have access to the Canada food rules. An older person living alone may not be independent in his need for diversion because he is unaware of the community resources (Golden Age Club, municipal library) at his disposal.

The initial data collection, even when done in great detail, is never finished, as new data are constantly emerging and others have been missed during the initial assessment. As the first step in the process, data collection is, however, as important as the subsequent steps and must be given the attention it deserves in the process of providing nursing care.

The initial data collection, sometimes called the nursing history, should be done as soon as possible in the client-nurse relationship. It is obvious that if the client is very tired or very upset, the interview should be postponed to a more opportune moment. In such a case the nurse will rely on her direct observation to make her initial assessment.

It is very difficult to remember all the information obtained from several clients unless that information has been noted in writing. Therefore, it is useful to develop an instrument known familiarly as the assessment tool. It serves not only the purpose of reminding the interviewer of the data she must collect, but as well provides her with a place to note the answers to her questions and to record any information volunteered by the client.

assessment tool

The type of assessment tool is a matter of personal preference. For some, a few key words for each fundamental need are all that is necessary, thus leaving the desired freedom to the interviewer; for others, it is more useful to have several questions prepared in advance for each fundamental need. In *neither* case must the nurse-interviewer be the slave of the assessment tool. It merely facilitates the systematic process, and the person who uses the tool must know it well and know also the conceptual model from which it derives. The usefulness of the tool lies in the fact that it helps the nurse obtain the information considered essential for her to plan and carry out nursing care.

If questions are prepared in advance, open questions are often considered more helpful than closed ones. "Can you tell me about your sleeping habits?" is more likely to solicit useful information than the closed question: "Do you sleep well?" It is understood, of course, that even the best-prepared questions should be altered according to individual circumstances. The words used to question a child are not always the same as those used to interview an adult. The nurse also changes her tone of voice and the form of the question in keeping with the reaction of the client, who may be visibly shy and ill at ease, or, on the contrary, very willing to talk about his needs.

When the client cannot answer questions, as in the case of a baby or an unconscious patient, the nurse-interviewer turns to the family. If the family is not present, or ill-disposed to answer questions, the nurse resorts to her direct observation and to the other sources of information. If data cannot be obtained, it is not because no data exist, but because circumstances make collection impossible at the moment.

It is of particular importance to understand that the assessment tool is derived from the conceptual model and not from a specific client population. The tool is built around the fourteen fundamental needs, indicating that every individual should be viewed holistically. The tool is not constructed strictly for cardiac patients or for psychiatric patients or for any other particular client group. The nursing assessment does not depend on the medical diagnosis, although the information it obtains will certainly be different *because* of that diagnosis. In some instances (*e.g.*, patients receiving home dialysis or industrial workers in a danger-filled environment), a page of supplementary questions may be added to the general assessment tool.

The complex art of interviewing and all the qualities necessary to be a successful interviewer are beyond the scope of this text. Suffice it to say that a helping relationship between client and nurse is extremely important.

Collecting the information necessary to help a client, in nursing as in other helping professions, requires a certain amount of time, and it has become trite to say that we do not have enough of that commodity. While it is true that time is very precious, it is always used in *some* way. If the nurse cannot find the time to collect the information that is essential to her, if she does not have time to take a nursing history before acting, what exactly is taking up her time? If she is not using her time to nurse, how is she using it?

It goes without saying that in an emergency situation all available personnel are mobilized in strictly life-saving procedures. At such times, the nurse willingly becomes the physician's assistant and may even, in special circumstances, act in his place. To do otherwise would be reprehensible. The nurse who finds herself constantly in the role of helping the physician in life-saving measures must, however, sometimes wonder if she is practising her own profession or someone else's.

A great many patients or health clients are not "emergency cases", and yet they expect and wish to have the help of the nurse. If that health professional claims to maintain or restore the client's independence in the satisfaction of his basic needs, she owes it to herself, and to the client, to take the time to assess that client's needs. The more clients she has to look after, the more she will want to save time by doing a nursing assessment at the beginning of the client-nurse relationship.

Bureau-Jobin and Pepin (1983) describe the long and painstaking process of developing an assessment tool and carrying out its initial testing. The questionnaire in the Appendix of this book is Pepin's translation and adaptation of that assessment tool.

In the description of their tool based on Henderson's frame of reference for nursing, Bureau-Jobin and Pepin (1983) point out that for each fundamental need, the open and closed questions cover the bio-physiological and the psycho-socio-cultural dimensions, the client's activities with regard to the need, and the changes in those activities because of his health problem. The nurse's observations are also included for each need.

Experimenting with the assessment tool was done in two community settings; clients had a wide variety of medical diagnoses. In the first setting, thirty clients of a home-care programme were interviewed twice: first by a community nurse using their regular assessment "guide", and secondly by a research colleague using the assessment tool (Bureau, 1981). The second setting was a different health centre where the home-care nurses used the assessment tool during a four-month period of adopting Henderson's way of looking at nursing (Pepin, 1980).

In the first setting, data collection interviews with the "guide" (53 items) took from 30 to 90 min with an average of 52 min;

those with the "tool" (72 items) lasted from 40 to 75 min for an average of 57 min. More than twice the amount of relevant information was obtained with the tool. Data of a psycho-socio-cultural nature were five times more abundant with the tool than with the guide.

When information had been collected using the tool, an average of 24.9 specific needs per client could be identified, compared with an average of 11.2 specific needs per client when the guide was used.

In the second setting, the nurses found that, even for clients they had known for some time, the assessment tool helped them to learn more about their clients, particularly from a psycho-socio-cultural point of view. However, the nurses found the tool long and they stated they were less comfortable with the questions related to the needs to communicate, to worship and to work so as to have a sense of accomplishment. The more the nurses became familiar with the tool, the more they felt at ease with the psycho-social dimensions of all the fundamental needs.

Bureau-Jobin and Pepin (1983) conclude that even the best assessment tool is useful only in the hands of a nurse who is not only familiar with the tool but who also, and more importantly, knows its underlying conceptual base.

interpretation of data

The information that has been obtained must be analysed and interpreted if it is to lead to effective intervention. Data that are not useful at subsequent steps of the systematic process should not be collected, for the client will only conclude that his privacy has been invaded for no reason. Having confided certain information to a nurse, the client has the right to believe that it will be put to good use.

In independence nursing, the analysis and interpretation of data, which is done with the client's participation, consists of three operations:

1. identifying specific needs

2. determining if they are satisfied independently or not
3. identifying the source of non-satisfaction for the unsatisfied needs.

A specific need is a particular or individual need; it is more restricted and more limited than a fundamental need, which is basic to all humans. For example, the need to keep the body clean is shared by all humans, sick or well; having a shower every morning, taking a bath twice a week, or washing one's hair every day are examples of personal or specific needs. (See chapter 8 for more details about the concept "need".)

Only after a specific need is identified is it possible to decide if it is satisfied independently or not. If the client satisfies the need on his own, the nurse must maintain that independence. If the need is not satisfied independently, the related source of non-satisfaction must be identified; the third operation consists in asking the question, "If not, why not?" If the need is not satisfied, is it because of a lack of strength (visual, intellectual, muscular, or cerebral), of will, or of knowledge?

In this way, a dependency problem in need-satisfaction is identified. A problem statement is made. (Some would say a nursing diagnosis is made. For more on nursing diagnosis, see chapter 14.)

Data interpretation does not mean determining the level of independence or the degree of satisfaction. Nursing research has not yet developed the measuring tools that might permit the establishing of degrees of dependency or levels of satisfaction.

As an example, let us imagine that Mr. Jones has just had abdominal surgery under general anaesthesia. In relation to his fundamental need to breathe, the nurse identifies two specific needs for Mr. Jones: (1) do breathing exercises for five minutes every hour and (2) cough and expectorate after each five-minute period. (These specific needs do not come from data collected from Mr. Jones, but from the nurse's knowledge of the effects of an anaesthetic on the respiratory tract and of the effects of an abdominal incision on thoracic movements.)

The specific needs are not satisfied; on the contrary, Mr. Jones seems to avoid risking even one deep breath.

The answer to the question, "If not, why not?" may be a lack of strength of the abdominal muscles. The source of non-satisfaction might also be a lack of knowledge about how to do the exercises; the preoperative teaching was not done or was not effective. A third possibility is that the source of Mr. Jones' dependency problem is insufficient motivation to do the exercises.

Three different problem statements can therefore be made. One, two or all three of them could be appropriate for Mr. Jones.

When a nurse is not able to identify specific needs proceeding from a given fundamental need, it is not because the client does not have any. Every client has fourteen basic needs and therefore has individual particularities related to each one. It may be that more time is required to establish a climate of confidence, or it may be that more data must be collected before specific needs can be identified together with their source of non-satisfaction.

In stressing the importance of the client's participation, the nurse not only shows her respect for him but also admits realistically that, with his help, she has a better chance of identifying real needs than if she acted unilaterally. The results can only be more satisfactory for both client and nurse.

In the interpretation of data, the nurse respects the plan of other professionals. From the information obtained from the client and from her own observations and experience, she may, for example, identify a specific need to drink a glass of fluid every two hours. If, however, the medical plan calls for a period of fasting in preparation for a diagnostic test, the need for extra fluids becomes, for the moment, a need to fast, and helping the patient remain fasting may call for more ingenuity than helping him to drink.

planning the intervention

A nursing intervention must now be planned that will help the client satisfy his specific need, in spite of his dependency problem, that is, in spite of his insufficiency of strength, will, or knowledge. Specific needs must be satisfied, if not by the client himself, then by the nurse's intervention.

Intervention, always of a complementing-supplementing nature, includes the focus of intervention, the mode of intervention and the intervention itself. If Mr. Jones does not do his breathing exercises because of a lack of strength of his abdominal muscles, the focus of intervention is the abdominal musculature, the mode of intervention is "reinforce", and the actual intervention could be to support the incisional area with a pillow during the exercises. As soon as possible, the nurse will show Mr. Jones how to support his incision himself.

If the need is not satisfied because of insufficient knowledge of how to do so, the intervention focus is Mr. Jones' knowledge, the intervention mode is "complete" or "add to", and the actual nurse's action could be to explain and demonstrate how to do the exercises. If Mr. Jones does not satisfy his need because he is not motivated enough, the focus of intervention is his motivation, the mode of intervention to "increase", and the nurse's activity to do the exercises with him and have him use a visual stimulant (such as displacing water with each forced expiration).

The six modes of intervention (the verbs used by Henderson to refer to the nurse's complementing-supplementing activities) are all additive. In many cases, they are therefore interchangeable. Knowledge may be increased, added to or completed; erroneous ideas can be replaced by more factual information. Strength (muscular, cerebral, etc.) may be reinforced, increased, replaced or substituted. Motivation may be reinforced or increased; since a person motivates or re-motivates himself, a nurse cannot replace his motivation or substitute her motivation for his. The modes are therefore not always interchangeable, but to argue, for example, that "completing knowledge" is more correct than "adding to knowledge" is to use time and energy that could be put to better use.

Adding to a client's strength may often mean reducing the opposing strength. A client may not be able to sleep because of the strength of his pain (or anxiety); he cannot sleep because he does not have the strength to overcome the opposing strength. The nurse who wants to increase the client's strength in relation to the pain's strength will attempt to reduce the latter; her actual intervention is on reducing the pain's strength. In the same way, the elderly client who must be moved to a new and strange environment may find he cannot walk as he has always done and as he needs to continue doing; he is unable to cope with a too-slippery floor, that is, he does not have the strength to combat the greater strength of the slippery surface. (There is no doubt that the client has the necessary knowledge and will to walk.) Increasing the client's strength means decreasing the opposing strength of the environment; the nurse's intervention of obtaining wall railings and a different floor covering will benefit a great many clients.

implementation

The fourth step of the clinical process, the carrying out of the planned intervention, is of great importance. A detailed data collection, a precise interpretation, and the most careful planning are all for naught if they are not followed by a competently executed action. Every step, of course, must be accompanied by a helping client-nurse relationship.

The various techniques, both manual and verbal, that make up the nurse's interventions are beyond the scope of this text.

evaluation

The fifth complex step in the complex process is evaluation. To appreciate this step, it is worthwhile recalling the desired consequences of independence nursing: the immediate one is need satisfaction while the mid-term or long-term consequences are increased client independence in need satisfaction or, in some cases, a peaceful death.

Evaluation is therefore the answer to the questions, "Are the specific needs satisfied?", "Is client independence increased?" and "Is the client living his last moments in dignity?". If the answers are negative, the steps of the systematic process must be examined in reverse order. Was the nurse's action carried out skilfully and competently and in a helping relationship? Was the correct action chosen? Perhaps an alternative complementing-supplementing strategy would be more effective. Was the source of difficulty correctly identified? Was the specific need realistic? Was the data collection complete enough to continue with the subsequent steps of the process?

Because the client's situation may change from week to week, from day to day, or even from hour to hour, new data must be constantly added to the initial collection. New information calls for the identification of new needs and all the subsequent steps of the process.

The systematic method constitutes the bridge between the abstract mental picture one has of nursing and the concrete interpersonal service one provides. The mental frame of reference is a way of conceptualizing nursing, while the systematic process is a way of proceeding; the latter is based on the former. The systematic method is a working instrument for practitioners and an educational tool for educators and students. The five steps of the process encompass another working instrument known as the *nursing care plan.*

nursing care plan

The written plan to be followed in the carrying out of care is composed of the second and third steps of the systematic process: interpretation of data and planning of intervention. In independence nursing, those steps are:

1. identification of the client's specific needs and of the source of their non-satisfaction
2. planning the focus and mode of intervention as well as the intervention itself, the supplementing-complementing action.

If the care plan is kept up to date, concise, and simple, it becomes an extremely useful means of written communication that contributes to the continuity of care as well as to more personalized care. In hospital nursing, the written care plan improves communications between day, evening and night nurses; each team finds important information on the care plan and adds new information to it. In home or community nursing, the written care plan re-acquaints the nurse with care objectives and other variables each time she renews contact with the client. As the systematic process is a dynamic method, so also the written care plan evolves continually with the changing needs of the client.

A written care plan may have various formats from the now familiar "Kardex" to the loose-leaf binder. Whatever the size and shape, the essential elements of a care plan are the individual needs of the patient and the planned nursing interventions. It must be remembered that a need is a requirement or a necessary activity; it is therefore written as the necessary client behaviour. The nurse's intervention is written as the nurse's suggested behaviour. A part of Mr. Jones' care plan would be as follows:

Specific need	**Supplementing-complementing action**
(necessary client activity)	(suggested nurse activity)
• do breathing exercises for 5 min q 1 h	• support incision with pillow

The foregoing is a care plan in its simplest possible form. For teaching purposes, particularly with beginning students, it may be useful to have a care plan of seven columns: fundamental need, specific need, satisfied independently (yes-no), source of non-satisfaction, focus of intervention, mode of intervention, nurse's action. The detailed steps must always be carried out mentally; learning to do so may be facilitated by writing them on a care plan of seven columns.

The written care plan, however simple or elaborate, is a plan to be followed and a projection of what is *to be* done or *to be* achieved. The report of what *has been done* is noted elsewhere.

Because one or more specific needs are identified for each of the fourteen fundamental needs, some evidently will have priority. To decide the order of importance of all the client's needs that require her assistance, the nurse will find Maslow's (1970) hierarchy of needs particularly helpful. In his conceptual framework of human motivation, Maslow describes physiological needs as the "most prepotent of all". When they are satisfied, safety needs emerge. Higher still in the hierarchy are love and belonging needs and when they are satisfied, needs for self esteem make themselves felt. At the top of the pyramid are the self-actualisation needs. Henderson & Nite (1978) refer specifically to Maslow's hierarchy.

The fourteen fundamental needs identified by Virginia Henderson fit into Maslow's hierarchy, although the level at which they may be placed is a question of individual differences. For one person, *the need to worship* corresponds to love and belonging needs, since the practice of his religion means sharing his faith with others of the same group. The same need to worship may belong at the level of self-actualisation in the case of a religious leader who fulfils himself in guiding others. In another example, *the need to communicate* may be, for some, at the level of self-esteem needs when the expression of opinions or feelings is a means of earning respect, status, or fame. For others, or indeed for the same person at another time, communicating may fit into the hierarchy at the level of love and belonging needs.

It may be useful to remember that following the method known as the systematic process does not lessen the importance of cooperating with medicine. Nurses will continue to carry out doctors' orders; that part of their work is clearly defined.

The independent part of nursing, that part which is "more than carrying out doctors' orders", must be made more explicit. Once that concept is clarified, the systematic process offers a means *by which* abstraction can be linked with reality.

The following chapter describes another systematic process—*the problem-solving method.*

chapter 5

the problem-solving method

The scientific process of problem-solving, widely used in nursing as well as in other disciplines, will be examined in this chapter.

Before exploring the steps of the process and its usefulness to nurses, the word "problem" must be defined. In the nursing literature, the word may be used one way in a research context and perhaps quite differently in a practice or education setting. Each writer seems to feel as confident as Humpty Dumpty did when he assured Alice that whenever *he* used a word, it meant exactly what he wished it to mean, no more, no less.

Popular usage of the word "problem" suggests something unpleasant or a difficulty to be overcome, although it is also used to signify a task to accomplish or a question to be answered. Webster's dictionary defines problem as "a source of perplexity, distress or vexation". In Abdellah's (1964) identification of twenty-one nursing problems presented by patients, the word corresponds to a nursing function, or a goal to achieve.

For the purposes of this text, the word problem is a difficulty to be reduced or removed.

The problem-solving method is used by many different professionals as well as by most everyone as they face and solve the large and small problems of daily living. As in the case of the systematic process described in the previous chapter, the problem-solving method is for some an instinctive way of proceeding. Francis (1967) describes five levels of problem-solving, ranging from the lowest, used by animals, to the highest, used by humans, and known as the *scientific method*. From infancy to old age, one attempts to overcome, either intuitively or in consciously organized fashion, the numerous difficulties of living, including physical discomfort, loneliness, and fear.

The helping professions apply themselves to solving problems in an organized and scientific manner; the members of the discipline are prepared to help clients overcome their difficulties. Not all professionals are competent to solve the same client problems, and new professions may be born to help with new problems and concerns. Each helping profession deals with the problems that are within its own area of competence and generally leaves to other professions problems that belong to their particular sphere of capability.

Just as the systematic process described in chapter 4 is highly useful, the scientific method for the solution of problems can also be used by nurses. Here too a similar question immediately comes to mind: "Which client problems are within the nurse's area of competence?" In other words, among the various difficulties that a client of the health services may present, which ones can the nurse, because of her particular preparation, solve better than another health professional?

Once again, the answer to the question is found in the nurse's conceptual framework. Following the one described in chapter 3, the client's problems that are within the scope of the nurse's capabilities are the client's problems of dependency in the satisfaction of his needs. Potential or actual dependency problems not only fall within the nurse's sphere of competence, but as a health professional she is *committed* to solving them—or preventing them.

Delineating in this way the nurse's "territory" allows her to cooperate efficiently with the other members of the interdisciplinary team, all of whom share the goal of improved health for the client. Because the nurse's contribution to the common goal is clearly defined, she will respect her co-workers' respective contributions and will accept the inevitable overlapping that occurs in a team approach. If the nurse is called upon to substitute temporarily for another member of the team, neither she, nor her colleague, nor the client, sees her as an instant expert in that area; the nurse's particular skill is *nursing*, and the difficulties she is especially prepared to handle are dependency problems.

The confusion in nursing terminology is well discussed by Bloch (1974); she points out that a *nursing* problem "... is a patient health problem which is expected to respond to the type of action or intervention carried out by a nurse, and a *medical* problem can be conceptualized as a patient health problem expected to respond to the type of action carried out by a physician." (p. 690)

The different steps of the problem-solving method vary somewhat from one writer to another.

Johnson (1970) identifies six steps:

1. encountering a problem or situation in which you discover a problem
2. assessing the problem or situation, that is, collecting and analysing the data in connection with it
3. identifying the exact nature of the problem
4. deciding a plan of action
5. carrying out the plan
6. evaluating the plan and the new situation

Coping with a difficulty in a methodical manner, such as the above, is appropriate for any kind of problem. This chapter is concerned only with the health problems of patients or clients and, more specifically, those known as nursing problems. The problems of nursing or of the nurse, such as personnel shortage and collective bargaining disputes, while very real and important, will not be discussed in this book.

The systematic process and the problem-solving method can now be compared and their similarities demonstrated.

Systematic process	Problem-solving method
1. data collection	1. encountering a difficult or distressful situation
2. interpretation of data	2. collecting and analysing the data connected with it

3. planning the intervention

3. identifying the exact nature of the problem

4. implementation

4. deciding a plan of action

5. evaluation

5. carrying out the plan

6. evaluating the action

The two proceedings are so similar that one is often taken for the other. Indeed, Bloch (1974) outlines a circular five-step "nursing process" where the second step is "definition of the problem." Either method defined above is useful to nurses; however, both must issue from a clear and precise conception of nursing.

One process may replace the other, or the two may complement each other.

The problem-solving method can be utilized either instead of or complementary to the systematic process. We shall now examine this statement in depth:

A. The problem-solving method instead of the systematic process

1. *Encountering a difficult situation:* when a person becomes a client of any health agency, it is entirely possible that he might be helped by a nurse. Such is not always the case; a health problem is not necessarily connected with a dependency problem in the satisfaction of basic human needs.

2. *Collecting and analysing the data connected with the difficulty:* in this step, information concerning the client's independence in his fourteen fundamental needs is obtained using the assessment tool. The analysis consists of identifying the specific or personal needs that derive from the fundamental needs and which the client cannot satisfy himself.

3. *Identifying the exact nature of the problem:* the precise form of dependency is now defined. The probable origin of the dependency is identified. It may be lack of strength, will, or knowledge. For example, instead of identifying a need in positive terms (*e.g.*, "begin to inject his insulin"), a dependency

problem is identified as "cannot inject his insulin because of insufficient knowledge" or "does not know how to inject his insulin." Instead of formulating in positive terms another patient's need to express his feelings about his prognosis, a problem is identified in negative terms: "does not, or cannot, express his feelings about his prognosis, because of diminished will or motivation to do so."

4. *Deciding a plan of action:* according to the conceptual model, the nurse's action is one of supplying what is lacking in strength, will or knowledge, so that the patient recovers his independence. In the preceding example, the nurse chooses the intervention mode "complete"; her plan of action is to complete the client's knowledge by teaching him the essentials of insulin injection by demonstrating the procedure or having the client practise the injection on an orange. In the situation where the client could not easily express his feelings, the nurse might choose the intervention mode "increase" and plan to increase the patient's motivation by demonstrating her readiness to listen, spending more time with the client, or being attentive to any attempt to discuss his prognosis in order to encourage and reinforce those attempts.

5. *Carrying out the plan.*

5. *Evaluating the plan:* is the one client more independent in injecting his insulin and the other in expressing his feelings? If not, must another plan of action be found, has the problem been correctly identified, or has the proper information been collected?

3. The problem-solving method complementing the system-tic process

Even as the systematic process is being carried out, difficulties may be encountered: the specific need defies identification, the identified need remains unsatisfied, or an effective intervention cannot be found. The difficulty can be examined and perhaps overcome by using the problem-solving method. The systematic process is continued meanwhile for the other needs, but the problem posed by one aspect of the process must be resolved.

As an example, we return to Mr. Jones. Let us suppose that his specific need to do breathing exercises every hour is not satisfied and the nurse is at a loss about how to improve the situation. In spite of all her efforts, Mr. Jones does not do his exercises and the recovery of his respiratory independence is therefore threatened. The specific need is correctly identified and seems realistic; the nurse's intervention must be at fault. It is clearly a case for the problem-solving method, in the hope of overcoming the difficulty as quickly as possible. The steps in this approach are:

1. the distressful situation is recognized

2. the collection of data connected with the situation encourages Mr. Jones to talk about his "refusal" to do his exercises and the nurse learns that the patient is afraid to breathe in deeply. She continues to explore the situation with Mr. Jones; he is not afraid of provoking pain on forced inspiration, nor is he apprehensive about bursting his sutures. What is causing his fear? He finally relates an unpleasant experience that happened to one of his friends in a personal growth workshop when, during breathing exercises, a forced inspiration had provoked great anxiety and an outburst of tears.

3. the exact nature of the problem is identified: Mr. Jones is afraid of an outburst of anxious tears if he takes a deep inspiration.

4. the plan of action is now to increase Mr. Jones' verbal expression of his fear and to substitute more realistic information about post-operative breathing exercises for the somewhat erroneous ideas he now has. The nurse's action is threefold:

   a. encourage Mr. Jones to speak of his fear
   b. remind him often of the reason for the deep-breathing—to help him cough and expectorate secretions
   c. use strictly physiological terms in coaching him, *i.e.* "breathe oxygen into your nostrils, now into your trachea into your bronchi and now into your lungs. Breathe out ..."

5. *Carrying out the plan:* the nurse proceeds as planned, assuring Mr. Jones that he can stop the exercises for a few moments if he becomes anxious.

6. *Evaluating:* Mr. Jones does his exercises every hour, for five minutes; he coughs and expectorates after each exercise period.

If the nurse's intervention is not effective, the problem-solving process must be maintained until the difficulty is overcome and the patient becomes more and more independent in the satisfaction of his individual needs.

Before leaving the subject of problem-solving, a word about a quite different point of view, one developed at first for physicians and now popular among nurses: Problem-Oriented Nursing or the Problem-Oriented System. Developed by Dr. Lawrence Weed, the Problem-Oriented Record assumes that the problem to be solved is the patient's problem and that the various health professionals all work toward solving that problem. Nurses who have adopted the method enthusiastically report that at long last there is one plan of care for the patient and his problem, rather than a nursing care plan and a medical plan (Woody & Mallison, 1973). Schell and Campbell (1972), in the first of two articles on Problem-Oriented Medical Records, also relate that the great advantage of the method is that it provides one approach, common to both physicians and nurses.

In yet another publication, doctors and nurses alike question the fact that "nursing has sought to break away from its subordinate position." Nurses' "flight from the role of handmaiden" poses a potential threat to the goal of comprehensive care (Woolley, 1974, p. 3). The authors recommend a team approach to patient problems. The problem list—a concise summary of the patient's problems—is a check list; nurses may identify and record problems "... and may consult the physician when they need assistance." (p. 15) Examples of problems are gastrointestinal bleeding, hypertension, and social isolation.

It seems clear that the way in which the problem-solving method is used depends directly on the conceptual framework to which one refers for the answer to the question: "What problems?" Nurses who see nursing as having the same social mission as medicine will apply themselves to solving the same problems as physicians. Those who, on the contrary, conceive nursing as having a specific role in health care, will attempt to solve the client's health problems that fall within their particular sphere of competence.

As demonstrated in the preceding chapters, nurses who consider their profession autonomous can choose to adopt a conceptual framework that clarifies nurses' singular contribution to health while at the same time underlining cooperation with other members of the interdisciplinary team in the best interests of the public.

chapter 6

the helping relationship

The purpose of this chapter is not to describe the helping relationship, since numerous authors from many different disciplines have done so; library shelves are well stocked with excellent books on interpersonal communication, the therapeutic relationship, and the interchange between the one who seeks help and the helper. The intent is rather to situate the helping relationship in the context of nursing care.

All of the helping professions are concerned with the relationship that exists between the client and the professional. The helping relationship is not exclusive to any one discipline. All the members of the health team are aware of the importance of establishing and maintaining a helping relationship; all wish to offer their help in an atmosphere of mutual confidence and open communication.

Nursing is no exception to the rule; the profession has long recognized the importance of the interpersonal relationship between patient and nurse. The helping relationship cannot, however, be used in nursing or applied to nursing as can the problem-solving method; the helping relationship is rather an integral thread of the very fabric of nursing, without which the nurse could never attain her particular goal.

The helping relationship is not, therefore, something that is unique to nursing, nor is it unique to nursing in any particular setting. It is, however, the *sine qua non* of effective nursing care. Whatever the conceptual model chosen, the helping relationship is indispensable.

But what is this all-important relationship? Although some writers discuss it only in a psychotherapeutic or psychiatric context, others indicate that a helping relationship is desirable every time one human being enters into contact with another, especially if one is perceived as a helper, *e.g.*, doctor, nurse, teacher, legal advisor, etc.

Obviously, the help offered by a legal advisor is not the same as that offered by a nurse. Each helper, pursuing the specific goal of his profession, offers his particular service in such a way that the client will perceive it as helpful. The nurse who seeks to restore her client's independence in the satisfaction of his needs will fulfil her complementary-supplementary role in such a way that the client will qualify the relationship between them a helpful one.

In a chapter entitled "The Interpersonal Relationship: The Core of Guidance", Rogers (1971) writes that in "professional work involving relationships with people—whether as a psychotherapist, teacher, religious worker, guidance counselor, social worker, clinical psychologist—it is the *quality* of the interpersonal encounter with the client which is the most significant element in determining effectiveness." (p. 85) If nursing may be included in the list of professional work that implies relationships with people, then it is the quality of the nurse-client encounter that is the most meaningful determinant in the effectiveness of nursing care.

While every encounter between two people is not necessarily a helping relationship, it seems that no meeting of humans can take place without some communication occurring. According to Watzlawick (1967), all behaviour is communication; no matter how one may try, one cannot *not* communicate. "Activity or inactivity, words or silence all have message value: they influence others and these others, in turn, cannot *not* respond to these communications and are thus themselves communicating." (p. 49) The implications for nursing, which often boasts of providing a twenty-four hour presence, are evident. In her many varied contacts with patients, the nurse will, ideally, communicate only messages of a helpful nature.

Perhaps because some authors emphasize a psychological approach while others stress physical and technical care, there is some tendency among nurses to think that while a helping relationship is important in some nursing situations, it can be dispensed with in others. Respect, kindness and understanding have always been highly valued in nursing. Yet the outward behaviour that reflects these inner attitudes is unfortunately not always observed in nurse-patient relationships. Who has not known at least one friend or relative who, as a patient, even while he recognized the technical efficiency of the nurses, complained bitterly that no one listened to him, nor understood him, nor treated him with respect? The charge that the public finds less kindness and courtesy among health professionals than from their most "impersonal" contacts, provides abundant food for thought for the "helping" professions.

This writer believes that all nursing care should be a demonstration of the helping relationship and that at all steps of the systematic process the nurse's behaviour should reflect the inner attitudes of a helper. For her nursing intervention to be effective, the nurse must remember the determining influence of the quality of her interaction with the client. To expect and demand this of her only underlines the fact that it is not easy to be a nurse. There is nothing simple about helping a fellow human being, and the nurse, no more than any other helper, cannot acquire a hundred per cent mastery of the fundamental attitudes essential to a helping relationship.

Many nurses, including Hein (1973), Orlando (1961), Peplau (1952), Travelbee (1966), and Ujhely (1968), have described the helping relationship that should exist between client and nurse. These valuable writings have been around for a long time, yet many nurses still seem to associate a helping relationship more with the nursing of psychiatric patients than with the care of others.

Few people are likely to dispute the fact that being a nurse can be difficult. Yet, if today's nurse claims equal status with other health professionals, as well as the accompanying salary, she can hardly exempt herself from the obligation of developing the attitudes that characterize a "helper." Not only must she make clear the nature of her contribution to societal health, she must also offer her service within a relationship that the client perceives as a helping one.

A relationship of some kind always exists between the client and the nurse. As do other health professionals, the nurse wants the relationship to be perceived by the client as a helping one, rather than an authoritarian or demeaning one, or a relationship he might have with a spouse, a close friend, or a business rival. A client-nurse relationship, however the client may qualify it, cannot *not* exist during every contact between the two. The relationship, in and of itself, is not an intervention to be carried out, for example, when other tasks have been completed. It is not something "to be done" at a certain time. The relationship *is*; the nurse must demonstrate by her words and actions the attitudes necessary for the client to perceive the relationship as "helping".

To pursue the systematic process effectively, a helping relationship is certainly necessary. In the first step of collecting information, unless a minimum of mutual confidence has been established, the client is apt to find questions about his elimination habits and health learning needs embarrassing indeed. The way the interview is conducted, and the manner in which the data are obtained, testify to the nurse's understanding and listening ability.

It is difficult to have the client participate in his care plan (the second and third steps of the process) if the nurse does not demonstrate some empathy and respect. The nurse indicates her confidence in the client by accepting his opinion, respecting his preferences, and allowing him as much choice as possible in his care.

The fourth step, the nursing action (a manual technique or a verbal intervention), can easily be perceived to be an intrusion of the patient's privacy unless it is accompanied by helping messages. At the fifth step, evaluation, the nurse's attentive listening and understanding are necessary if she is to judge the satisfaction of needs and an increase in independence.

We are once more faced with the evidence that to be a nurse, that is, to help another, is a demanding profession. Nursing is known as one of the helping professions. Understanding and respecting the client imply, of course, that the nurse understand and respect herself, as a person and as a nurse. If self-knowledge and self-respect are acquired throughout an entire lifetime, beginning at birth, the knowledge and respect associated with being a nurse are first acquired through professional education. The following chapter discusses that education.

In summary, the helping relationship, while common to several professions, is essential for effective nursing. Whatever professional goal the nurse chooses to pursue—independence according to Henderson (1966), adaptation according to Roy (1984), or behavioural equilibrium according to Johnson (Riehl & Roy, 1980), to name only three—she will strive to imprint all her professional activities with the mark of helping communication.

Table: Interactions among the helping relationship, conceptual model, and systematic process.

HELPING RELATIONSHIP	CONCEPTUAL MODEL	SYSTEMATIC PROCESS

Empathy
Respect
Understanding
Warmth
Listening
Confidence
	Assumptions
	Values
	Units: Goal
	      Client
	      Social role
	      Source
	      of difficulty
	      Intervention
	      Consequences
		Collection of data
		Interpretation
		Planning
		Implementing
		Evaluation

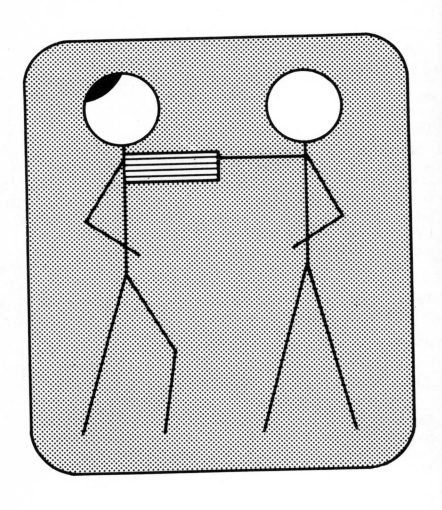

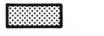 Helping Relationship    Conceptual Model   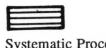 Systematic Process

chapter 7

independence nursing: education, practice, research

The adoption of Henderson's conceptual model means that nursing education, practice and research will be based on that conception of the profession.

nursing education

Only one aspect of such a vast and complex subject will be discussed. The "how" of teaching is influenced, but only indirectly, by one's conception of the subject to be taught—nursing. Some very important aspects of nursing education, such as learning theories, teaching methods, the preparation of teachers and so forth, are beyond the scope of this chapter.

The mental picture that one has of nursing does, however, influence directly the "what" of teaching, *i.e.*, educational goals and objectives, and the content of the program itself. The conceptual model chosen makes explicit the very nature of nursing; it thus provides, at each stage of a nursing programme, important elements of the answers to such questions as "Whom do we want to prepare? For what role are we preparing the student? What must she know in order to fulfil that role?"

In independence nursing, the curriculum is planned to prepare a health worker capable of maintaining and restoring the client's independence in the satisfaction of his needs. To do so, the student learns a complementary-supplementary role, discussed earlier in this book. Details vary, of course, with the educational level of the students and objectives of the programme.

The *official content* of a curriculum based on Virginia Henderson's conception of nursing will now be examined. First, however, official content must be distinguished from *unofficial content*, an equally important part of any curriculum.

Unofficial content, sometimes referred to as "process as content", covers everything that is learned in an educational programme without being taught. Students can learn to be passive without ever taking a course in passivity; they can learn to dislike reading without ever signing up for a course in how to hate reading. In much the same way, nursing students may learn that their future role as a health professional defies all attempts at definition even though there is no course in the programme about lack of identity. In a more positive line of thought, students can learn to be enthusiastic and to ask questions without studying the art of being enthusiastic and asking questions. Students in a nursing programme can learn to value their specific contribution to the community's health without necessarily studying self-assertion as a member of the health team. Students "get the message" even though teachers do not consciously articulate the message (Postman & Weingartner, 1969).

The *official content*, that which is formally recognized and actually taught, is usually divided into two parts; nursing content and content that comes from related disciplines. Again, the proportion of each depends on the level of the programme and the previous preparation of the students.

The requirements of professional corporations and of government guidelines may impose certain obligations on curriculum planners concerning nursing and non-nursing content. However, such requirements, sometimes perceived as constraints, are developed by nurses or at least approved by them. Nurses are necessarily influenced in their decisions by their way of looking of nursing, whether their conception of nursing is clear and explicit or blurred and ambiguous.

It is important to note that the nursing programme is *based on* the conception of nursing. The conceptual model is not *taught*, in the sense that it is subject matter among other subjects to be taught. The conception of nursing on which the programme is based will' certainly be *learned*, but because it permeates all nursing content. Students enter a programme (college or university) to learn to be a nurse. Before they arrive, their nurse educators have chosen a conception of nursing as a basis for programme content: Stevens (1979) insists that teachers must have a clear conception of nursing before they attempt to teach it. MacQueen (1974) asks how anyone who does not have a clear mental image of nursing can teach people to be nurses.

In a programme based on Henderson's vision of nursing, students will learn independence nursing—its assumptions, values, and major units. They will learn that independence nursing is Henderson's conception of nursing. (They may know that a neighbouring school's programme is based on Johnson's or on Roy's conception of the discipline.) But no course outline will ever include "Henderson's model" as content. The model is not taught; it is nursing that is taught.

Related or non-nursing content is chosen according to the conceptual model for nursing. Because of the complexity of each fundamental need, knowledge of anatomy, physiology, pathology, psychology, sociology, anthropology, etc. is essential for independence nursing. Knowledge of health and ecology is equally important. Non-nursing content may include philosophy, the history of nursing, statistics, and many other courses.

Nursing content will include the concepts of wholeness, need, independence, need satisfaction, motivation, strength, and knowledge. The fundamental needs of well people from premature birth to old age will be studied in detail before the same needs are examined in relation to a variety of health problems. The systematic process will be completed theoretically for groups of patients before the student undertakes the process in the clinical field. The helping relationship will also be seen theoretically before clinical experiences begin.

The teaching of nursing content depends on the available knowledge in the human and biological sciences. Whether it comes from biochemistry, endocrinology, psychology or philosophy, current scientific knowledge is essential to the study of nursing as indeed it is to any other health discipline. Notions of touch, of grief and grieving, of pain and anxiety, or of death and dying are important for a nurse because they affect the client's independence in need satisfaction; whether the knowledge comes from nursing, from medicine or from theology, it is useful to nursing.

Nursing content is divided into theoretical and practical courses. The *practical* aspect will now be discussed. It consists of technical procedures (taught in the classroom and in the laboratory) and clinical experiences in various settings.

The "art" of nursing has traditionally occupied a place of honour in the eyes of both practitioners and educators. Procedures and techniques were perhaps given too much importance in educational programmes at a time when nursing was seen chiefly as the accomplishment of well-defined tasks and the carrying-out of doctors' orders. Later, as some nurses tried to emphasize other important aspects of patient care, techniques were given second or third priority and were considered, at least by some, as a necessary evil or something to be delegated to auxiliary personnel.

With today's conceptual models for nursing, which make explicit the profession's goal, role, and other parameters, techniques are restored to (for some, maintained in) their rightful place as an important aspect of nursing; not as an end in themselves, but as a means of achieving a specific goal. Techniques are an essential part of a complementary-supplementary role, a means of assisting the client in those activities that he would perform himself if he had the necessary strength, will, and knowledge. Techniques are one way of pursuing the ideal and limited goal: the client's independence in need satisfaction.

Technical procedures, traditional or modern, are simply part of a larger framework. For example, the time-honoured bed bath is a way to help the client satisfy his need for cleanliness and the sterile dressing is a means of satisfying the patient's need to avoid the danger of infection. Communication techniques are learned in order to help the client express his needs, to do a nursing assessment, and to maintain a helping relationship.

Certain procedures constitute a privilege for the nurse—a privilege that is denied to certain other members of the health care team. For example, as a form of non-verbal communication, touch is particularly eloquent; such comforting techniques as the back-rub, the sponge-bath and the change of position provide the nurse with frequent occasions to establish physical contact with her patient. As well as the physical comfort given, the time spent in such care can be used to explore less tangible aspects, such as the patient's anxiety or his need to confide in an understanding person. Techniques may therefore serve two purposes: the immediate comfort that follows and, equally important if not more so, the increased opportunity for the communication that is part of a helping relationship. Of great importance, of course, is the obligation to carry out, with kindness and efficiency, both comfort-giving procedures and pain-inflicting treatments.

Other techniques, such as the taking of vital signs, are learned in order to carry out doctors' orders and thus cooperate with the medical team. Our long tradition of a 24-hour presence in the hospital setting and of watching over the patient is not soon to disappear; the nurse's careful observations often contribute to the medical diagnosis and changes in medical treatment. Teaching such techniques to students not only assures interdisciplinary cooperation but also affords more possibilities for identifying the patient's individual needs as they emerge.

Periods of clinical experience are an important part of most professional programmes and have always been highly valued in schools of nursing; the proportion of "theory" and "practice" depends on the educational level of the programme. From an era when nurses were prepared almost entirely in a practice setting, we have come to a time of more theoretical and scientific programmes. While it is true that the useless repetition of overly learned techniques and the lack of coordination between classes and clinical experience are clearly not educational, it is also true that well-planned experiences in a variety of settings are very pedagogical and helpful. For a helping profession that places such a high value on inter-personal relationships and effective communication, it seems only logical that a nursing programme will provide students with opportunities for contact with clients in the home, hospital, or other setting.

The conceptual model indicates the nature of the clinical experiences. Progressing from the simple to the complex, the clinical instructor chooses the student's experiences according to the client's independence. The choice may be made on the basis of the patient's state of health. In general, for example, people with a skin problem are less dependent in satisfying their fundamental needs than are unconscious patients, and ambulatory patients are more independent than bed-ridden ones. The contrary may, however, prove true and those who, at first glance, seem quite independent have, in reality, dependency problems. The choice of clinical experiences is thus a time-consuming and demanding task for the teacher. The choice may also be suggested by the developmental stage; newborn infants are usually more independent than premature babies, but less so than adults.

The goal of clinical experiences is to provide the student with opportunities to help a client recover his independence in satisfying his needs. During her various experiences in different settings, the student will use the systematic process in the care of the comatose, the cardiac, and the woman in childbirth; she will attempt to solve dependency problems of leukemic, mentally ill, and post-operative patients; she will develop the attitudes of the helping relationship with the dying, with accident victims, and with diabetics, and she will learn her complementary-supplementary role with the aged, the newborn, and with adolescents. She will thus have contact with a multitude of health problems and in a variety of socio-economic situations. Her educational preparation is not organized around disease or pathology, but around potential or actual dependency problems.

The use of scientific knowledge as a base for nursing education depends on the educational level. The longer the programme, the more time there is for the student to acquire more knowledge, to learn creative and innovative ways of fulfilling her complementary-supplementary role, to identify subtle and complex needs, and to become skilful in establishing, maintaining, and terminating a helping relationship.

At the master's level, the thinking of Virginia Henderson can be the basis of a curriculum to prepare specialists in nursing practice, education and research, and also specialists in the administration of any of those fields. The clinical specialist would be an expert in independence. She might choose to specialize in maintaining or restoring independence in leukemic children, neurological patients, or clients from a given socio-economic group. The clinical nurse specialist might also choose to specialize in the satisfaction of one or several needs, such as the need to learn or to sleep and rest. The concept of independence in the fourteen fundamental needs would be the basis of all specialties, thus making a distinction between medical and nursing specialization. "If nursing is conceived of differently, why do we piggyback on medicine's emphasis when we specialize?" (Rogers, 1973, p. 3)

The graduate level is also the moment of choice for a comparative study of various conceptual models for nursing and the time to experiment with their consequences for education, practice and research. In a doctoral programme in nursing, students may use the concept of independence in need satisfaction as the basis of research for the development of nursing science.

The mental image of nursing therefore affects all levels of nursing education. Care must be taken, however, to avoid dividing up the fourteen needs among the various levels. Educators must *never* attribute certain needs to one programme, and reserve others for a higher-level programme. Since the client is conceptualized as a whole, to separate him into pieces would be an abuse, rather than a use, of the writings of Virginia Henderson. The most highly specialized of clinical nurse specialists should not lose sight of the client's wholeness and of his independence in the satisfaction of all his needs.

The conceptual model relates, at least indirectly, to the methods of teaching nursing. If the teacher wants the student to help the client to independence, the teacher should allow as much independence as possible to the student; the instructor will intervene, in the classroom and in the clinical setting, in accordance with the learning needs of the student. The teacher's efforts to be consistent and practise what she preaches will have an impact on all the unofficial content. For example, if she wants her student to listen to the patient, the teacher must listen to the student, and if the student is to learn respect for her clients, she herself must feel respected by her teachers.

In summary then, a complete and explicit conception of nursing, Henderson's or another's, gives direction to educators for the preparation of practitioners.

nursing practice

The conceptual model for nursing offers the same directions to the practitioner. In whatever setting chosen (community nursing, hospital nursing, social, family, home nursing), the nurse pursues the goal of independence for the client and assumes a complementary-supplementary role.

Chapters 3, 4, 5, 6, 8, 9, 10, 11 and 12 of this book touch on various aspects of nursing practice. Whatever the client's age or medical diagnosis, the problems that the nurse is prepared to handle are dependency problems in need satisfaction. Independence nursing is a helpful professional service for individuals, families or groups.

The evaluation of the quality of nursing care (quality assurance) is linked to the quality of practitioners. Do they have a clear mental image of what quality care should be? Is their social mission clear? Is their professional goal specific? At the moment, nurses are not required to have answers to such questions in order to obtain a licence to practise, or to have that licence renewed annually. While some nurses might protest the imposition of such criteria, others might welcome the obvious compliment: nursing *is* a specific service, one that can be presented in clear and explicit terms.

The practitioner will, of course, continue to carry out physician's orders. She may, however, question any new delegation of tasks, from whatever source, in order to give more time to her own professional activities so that her time will be entirely occupied by independence *nursing*; to be a nurse does not mean agreeing to be unit secretary, laboratory technician, or surrogate pharmacist.

Whether administrator of nursing service, bedside nurse, team-leader or clinical specialist, the practitioner in any work setting (community, home, hospital, etc.) carries out the social mission of contributing to the public's improved health by working toward greater client independence in need satisfaction.

nursing research

Although research methods and measuring tools used by nurse-researchers may come from other disciplines, the problems that constitute *nursing* research, rather than medical or sociological research for example, come from the nurse's mental picture of her own profession. To contribute to the advancement of nursing science, to build up a body of nursing knowledge and to develop nursing theories, the researcher explores avenues that are suggested to her by her conception of nursing.

The administrators of research funds, as well as the researchers themselves, choose to invest their time and energy in a certain problem because it is a nursing problem. In making that decision they are necessarily influenced by their concept of nursing, since it seems quite impossible not to have an idea of what nursing is, however vague that idea may be. Repeated and controlled studies of nursing problems can lead to useful conclusions and generalizations which, in turn, may provide researchers with the descriptive terms distinctive to nursing that are essential for theory construction.

Henderson's conceptual model is a useful starting point for researchers committed to independence nursing and the advancement of the discipline. A body of nursing knowledge could be built up from careful scrutiny into areas of concern for practice and education: the measuring of independence, of need satisfaction; the complementing of strength, will and knowledge; the specific needs of certain patients (the aged, the cognitively impaired, patients on chemotherapy, etc.); the dependency problems of certain patients; the termination of complementary-supplementary actions; the effects of pain, stress, grieving, etc. on independence in need satisfaction, on wholeness.

Independence nursing research is also discussed in chapter 13. When educators, practitioners and researchers, in various different settings, base their teaching, nursing care and research on Henderson's model, the latter can be evaluated using Johnson's (1974) criteria of social significance, congruence and utility. As in the evaluation of any conceptual model, the service that is based on Henderson's way of looking at nursing must be significant to the client's health and must correspond to his expectations; the model must also be a useful conceptual base for a nursing curriculum, for planning nursing care, and for identifying research problems.

If nurses do not make clear their singular contribution to society's health, they can hardly be surprised if they do not have the credibility and the political power that they would so like to have. If the words and actions of educators, practitioners, and researchers do not reveal a clear conception of nursing's distinct social mandate, nurses may not deserve to wield the political power or to enjoy the credibility of other health professionals.

The chart on page 65 illustrates the influence of nursing's conceptual base on education, practice and research.

It is nursing practice that justifies our claim to being a professional discipline (a helping profession, a practice discipline). Nursing education prepares students for practice; nursing research seeks to improve that practice and to develop theories that will provide the knowledge required for it. According to Stainton, Rankin & Calkin (1989), practice "is the *raison d'être* of nursing, research the tool for knowledge development, and education the medium through which the knowledge of practice is made available" (p. 20).

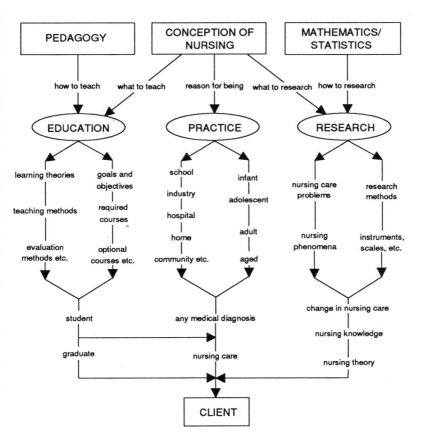

chapter 8

need and independence

This chapter discusses two concepts that are often, at least in some contexts, seen as being mutually exclusive. Popular use of the words seems to indicate that a person who has needs is in some way dependent, while the one who has no needs is independent. In the context of independence nursing, "need" and "independence" are so defined that they are entirely compatible.

need

In chapter 3, it was pointed out that need signifies requirement. The nurse's client is conceptualized as a complex whole made up of fourteen needs that are fundamental to all humans, whether they are well or suffering from a health problem. In other words, the person-as-client has fourteen necessary activities or requirements; the complexity of the human being is represented by fourteen fundamental imperatives or basic exigencies. The satisfaction of each need is essential to the person's wholeness.

Several nurse authors (Orlando, 1961; Roy, 1984; Watson, 1979) define need as a requirement. In an education context, Nadeau (1981) lists various possible definitions of need: lack, force, motivation, tension, desire, exigency, deficiency. A physician who states that a human being has twelve fundamental needs (examples are dignity, freedom, imagination) points out that a need is fundamental because it is a necessity for the individual (Dunn, 1959). Dictionaries offer a variety of meanings for the word "need": requisite, that which is necessary, requirement, necessity. The same dictionaries confirm that need is also defined as a "lack".

In this book, "need" is defined as requirement or necessity. The nurse's client is not a complex whole made up of fourteen deficiencies or "lacks", but, rather, a complex whole made up of fourteen requirements or exigencies. Five of the fundamental needs identified by Henderson (1966) are also known as vital needs: to breathe, eat and drink, eliminate body wastes, sleep and rest, and maintain body temperature. The fourteen needs are therefore not all essential to life; they are, however, all essential to the person's wholeness, completeness. The importance given to each need varies between individuals and, even for one person, the importance attached to any one need varies at different times. The priority of needs according to Maslow's hierarchy has been discussed in chapter 4.

The fourteen basic needs identified by Henderson (1966) have been described by other authors as the fourteen components of nursing care (Furukawa & Howe, 1980). This seems to be a departure from Henderson's notion that the fourteen needs are basic to the nurse's client; it is the satisfaction of those fourteen needs, in all their dimensions, that maintains the client's wholeness.

Roper *et al.* (1980) declare that the components of nursing are four in number: twelve activities of living, prevention, the nurse's comfort activities, and the nurse's dependent activities. For Roper *et al.*, the twelve activities of living, common to all humans, are situated on an independence-dependence continuum.

The components of nursing care, as described in this book (chapter 6) are the client (with his fourteen needs), the nurse (with her conceptual base and her systematic method), and the client-nurse relationship. In other words, the components of nursing care are three: the client, the nurse, and the relationship between them.

As stated in chapter 3, each basic need is, in itself, complex, with biological, physiological, psychological, social and cultural dimensions. The nurse who conceptualizes her client as a complex whole with fourteen basic requirements, considers that her contribution to health is the maintaining and restoring of client independence in the satisfaction of his specific needs that proceed from the fourteen fundamental needs of all persons.

The fourteen basic requirements of each person do not cease to be requirements when they have been met; the fundamental needs continue to be needs even when they have been satisfied. The satisfaction of the need to communicate, for example, does not abolish the human requirement to express one's ideas and feelings; the satisfaction of the need to learn does not cancel the human requirement to appease one's curiosity and slake one's thirst for knowledge. On the contrary; the satisfied need may no longer be felt so intensely, but its continued satisfaction is integral to the person's wholeness. At the end of a large and delicious meal, a person may remark that he will never be hungry again, that he will not "need" to eat again. However, that same person knows full well that the requirement to eat and drink has not disappeared.

As with other needs, the necessity to eat and drink is extremely complex. The "what", "when", and "how" of eating and drinking are often determined by the psycho-socio-cultural dimensions of the need and may be unrelated to any bio-physiological imperatives. One has only to consider a special meal to celebrate a particular occasion where the satisfaction of only the bio-physiological aspect of eating and drinking would be tantamount to non-satisfaction of the need; the "wholeness" of the person insists on particular dishes, special guests, and on numerous details of time, atmosphere, and liquid accompaniment. Spiritual or philosophical aspects, such as the sharing of bread, the offering of hospitality, and the expression of support and sympathy may be equally important on occasion.

A need, defined as requirement or necessity, must be distinguished from a "wish" or a "habit". The person who has the habit of drinking twenty cups of coffee a day may say that he "needs" that much coffee in order to get through his working day. Current knowledge indicates that so much caffeine is harmful to the human body; it follows that the person's specific need, derived from the fundamental need to eat and drink, cannot be to drink twenty cups of coffee a day. The person has the habit of drinking twenty cups daily; he wants to drink that amount; he has perhaps even developed a physiological and psychological dependency on caffeine, but he does not *need* twenty cups a day: that amount is not a *necessity*. The same person, aware that the habit is harmful to his health, may agree with the nurse that his specific need, in the area of eating and drinking, is to reduce the number of cups of coffee. He may realize that he drinks so much coffee because he sleeps poorly, and that he sleeps poorly because of personal and professional worries. Thus, the specific need to reduce his caffeine intake is closely related to other specific needs that flow from the fundamental needs to communicate, to rest and sleep, to learn and to avoid dangers. The client is always seen as a complex "whole"; to limit consideration to only one need, or to only one dimension of a need, is to deny the complexity of the client's wholeness.

The reasoning that led to the identification of a specific need to reduce caffeine intake may one day become invalid. If scientific knowledge should ever indicate that large amounts of caffeine are beneficial to the human organism, then our ideas on the subject will have to be revised. In the same way as other health professionals, nurses depend upon available scientific knowledge; our practice nay change with each new discovery in the human and biological sciences, whatever discipline claims the discovery. The fourteen fundamental needs of all humans may conceivably remain unchanged; our ideas about the specific needs that flow from them will change, however, with the evolution of scientific knowledge. One has only to consider the post-partum or post-operative patients of fifty years ago and their fundamental need to move. The fundamental requirement has not changed, but the specific needs that derive from it are very different today.

Another example will demonstrate the difference between a need and a habit in the context of independence nursing. A client may talk of his "need" for cigarettes, for alcohol, or for some other drug. The statement will be greeted with indulgence or irritation, depending on the person who hears him. From a health promotion perspective, the statement is understood as an inclination, a habit or a desire to smoke, to drink or to escape by taking other drugs. Certain habits, however much they may be entrenched in human behaviour, cannot be considered "needs", since they do not proceed from the person's fundamental requirements. In other words, there are human habits that, while they are understandable and, in some cases, quite tolerable, cannot be referred to as necessities. For the client, his harmful habit may be so important to him that he considers it absolutely necessary, even vital; for the nurse committed to independence nursing, an activity that is harmful to a person's health is not, strictly speaking, a *need*. (If the nurse were to accept it as a need, she would then have to make sure that it was satisfied, if not independently by the client, then through her intervention.)

Returning to the example of smoking, current knowledge tells us that nicotine is harmful to the pulmonary and cardio-vascular functions. Smoking, a habit that even today is still considered socially acceptable by some people, does not proceed from any fundamental need; not the need to breathe, nor the need to sleep and rest, nor the need to eliminate body wastes. For some people, of course, smoking is a *relatively* harmless habit. The intent here is not automatically to condemn the person who smokes, nor to identify an immediate need to suppress the habit. Attempts at moralizing or at converting the client to the professional's opinions are not always effective methods. What is important for the nurse is to avoid confusing "need" and "habit". A distinction will be made later between "need" and "means".

The requirements that make up the "whole"—the bio-psycho-social being—are not compatible with activities that are harmful to that being. Thus, in a health context, the wish or the longing to attempt suicide is not a specific need derived from the fundamental need to communicate. Nor is the compulsive habit of washing one's hands every ten minutes a specific need arising from the fundamental one to keep the body clean. The distinction between a need (which must be satisfied if the person's wholeness is to be maintained) and a whim, habit or caprice (which is harmful to the person's wholeness) is not always easy; the nurse must call upon considerable scientific knowledge as well as on her experience and her moral and professional conscience. She also refrains from imposing her own values on the client; the last word is always his, and he may choose to discard the professional's opinion.

All health professionals may eventually be faced with the dilemma of deciding just how far they can and should go in their attempts to convince a client to adopt a more healthy life style. The nurse is no exception. Conscious of her obligation to help the client make the best choice for himself, at that particular time in his life, the nurse may be called upon to make extremely difficult decisions. Her respect for the client's freedom to choose will help her avoid two extremes: on the one hand, to impose, or try to impose, her own values on the client and, on the other hand, to disavow all responsibility toward him.

The nurse who wishes to avoid those two extremes will remember that the client-nurse relationship, the quality of which determines the effectiveness of nursing care, is a most influential component of nursing. The quality of that relationship is, of course, the responsibility of both parties; it is, however, the nurse who demonstrates, by her words and actions, that she has the attitudes of a helper (empathy, active listening skills, etc.). When a conflict arises between nurse and client about the latter's specific needs, the nurse's emotional maturity will stand her in good stead, as will many other qualities, including a healthy dose of humility!

It may happen that certain habits are indeed needs. A person's habit of drinking a glass of milk every day and of sleeping six hours every night derive from two fundamental needs: to eat and drink, and to rest and sleep. The habits are necessary to the person's wholeness. They correspond to current knowledge about the requirements of the adult organism (although not at all to knowledge about a baby's requirements). They are indeed specific needs.

In the second step of the systematic method (*i.e.*, the nursing process) the nurse identifies, with the client's participation, the latter's specific needs. Each specific need must meet three criteria:

1. it flows from a fundamental need

2. it is an individual necessity (its satisfaction is required for the client's wholeness)
3. it is compatible with current scientific knowledge.

As well as respecting the three criteria, it is helpful, from a practical point of view, to formulate the specific need using an active and observable verb. Passive forms, such as "need to be taught ...", "need to be turned", or "need to be reassured" seem to make the client himself passive—someone to be acted upon. The active forms, such as "to learn ...", "to change position", and "to express his concerns" put the focus on the client's activities.

A specific need expressed in observable terms makes it easier to continue with the second step of the systematic process: is the need satisfied independently and, if not, why not? Thus, "drink 200 cc of liquid every two hours" is preferable to "increase hydration" or "increase fluid intake". "Eat a green vegetable every day" is observable, while "increase consumption of calcium" is not.

The use of active and observable verbs helps keep in mind that the client's fourteen fundamental needs are activities. For example, the fundamental needs are not "oxygenation" and "nutrition" but, rather, "to breathe normally" and "to eat and drink". A person's oxygenation and nutrition are extremely complex and involve the integrity of the vascular network, the permeability of the cell membrane, the blood's oxygen-carrying capacity, and many other operations that are not directly under the nurse's responsibility. What is directly amenable to the nurse's intervention is the activity of breathing, of eating and drinking.

The use of active and observable verbs also helps to avoid identifying desired emotions or feelings. The fundamental need is not "to feel useful" but "to work in such a way that ...". The accent is on the observable activity. With regard to feelings, most people would probably agree that the most important human needs include "to love and be loved", "to be happy", and "to have a positive self-esteem"; those very agreeable sentiments are not incompatible with independence nursing. The fourteen needs identified by Henderson are activities that are amenable to the nurse's intervention; the satisfaction of those needs will go a long way toward the client's feelings of being loved and useful, but the nurse's intervention is not directly on the emotion. When a client cannot, on his own, satisfy his needs to eat and drink, to keep clean, to eliminate body wastes, to communicate, to learn and indeed all the fundamental needs, the complementing-supplementing interventions of the nurse will contribute directly to their satisfaction; they will also contribute indirectly, but importantly, to maintaining or increasing the client's self-esteem and to other positive feelings. The absence of the nurse's complementing-supplementing certainly seems to contribute to the client's low self-esteem and other negative feelings.

Identifying a specific need may call for a distinction between the client's "need" and his "means" of satisfying it. (The nurse's means, that is, her complementing-supplementing interventions, are not discussed here.) A very effective means of satisfying a need, if it is not harmful to the client's health, may in time become one of his needs. For example, from an elderly man's fundamental need to communicate springs the specific need to talk to his only son every week. The means of doing so, visiting his son in person, becomes impossible because of the son's move to a distant city. A new means of satisfying the need, writing a letter, in turn becomes unrealistic because of increasing pain and limitations related to the aged man's arthritis. The need to communicate with his son remains. A new means, the long-distance phone call, becomes, with time, a precise way to formulate the need: telephone each week to his son. The nurse's intervention will be required, but the need will be satisfied.

Another client may identify, from his basic need to eliminate body wastes, a specific need to have a bowel movement every second morning. His means of stimulating peristalsis, drinking a glass of warm water on arising, is so effective that it becomes a specific need proceeding from his fundamental requirement to eat and drink: "drink a glass of warm water every morning" is now a necessity for his independence. In this way, a means of satisfying one need (to eliminate) is a specific need deriving from another (to eat and drink). The fourteen needs that make up the whole are closely linked. For example, a specific need to sleep with three pillows may derive from three fundamental needs: to breathe, maintain posture, and avoid dangers. It is not important to argue that the specific need should be classified under one or the other of the three fundamental needs; what is important is that the need be satisfied. For yet another client, the specific need to continue public speaking (despite a health problem) may proceed from one of several fundamental needs: to communicate, to work in such way that there is a sense of accomplishment, and to act in accordance with spiritual or religious beliefs.

To return to the example of the early-morning glass of warm water, it may be, for another client, not a specific need, but merely a means suggested by the nurse to supplement peristaltic strength; if it is not effective, another means will be sought. The client may find that an effective means of satisfying his need is to take a nightly laxative. This means, with its long-term harmful effects, is not compatible with current knowledge; it cannot, therefore, be a need. A laxative may be a temporary means; the intent here is not to condemn laxatives, but to make a distinction between "need" and "means".

A need is fundamental when it is a requirement of all human beings, well or unwell; Henderson has identified fourteen. A need is said to be specific, or particular, or individual, when it is a necessity or requirement that is not universal. A specific need, however, is not so individual that it is a need of only one person; it may be shared by many people. Particularly in the bio-physiological dimensions of the fundamental needs, a specific need may be common to a group of clients (premature babies, paraplegics, the elderly). A specific need that is shared by three or by sixty people is no less a necessity for each of those three, or each of those sixty people, and must be satisfied, if not by the person himself, then by the nurse's intervention.

Because certain specific needs are shared by a group of patients, "standard" care plans can sometimes be written.

Because not all specific needs are shared, an "individual" care plan is always necessary. Even when a specific need is shared by many, it is unlikely that the nurse's complementing-supplementing interventions will be the same for all, for the source of non-satisfaction may vary within the group.

Before concluding the discussion of needs, mention must be made of the needs of a small child. The earlier distinction between wanting and needing does not necessarily apply when the nurse's client is a baby. Developmental psychology has long affirmed that a baby's wishes are his needs; the newborn wants only that which he really needs. It would seem that adults, including nurses, can confidently trust the wisdom of the little one to want—and to choose—those things that are necessary to him. To the tired parent, of course, the baby's desires (needs) may seem to be caprices or whims: wanting to be held, wanting to breast-feed at irregular intervals, wanting attention at inconvenient moments. In a healthy context, the baby thus succeeds beautifully in satisfying his needs, in getting what he requires for his own development and therefore maintaining his wholeness.

Faced with the complexity of human needs accompanied by constantly evolving knowledge, the nurse's social mandate is a demanding one: maintain and restore client independence in the satisfaction of his specific needs that derive from the fundamental needs of all humans.

independence

Dictionaries define independence as the absence of dependence (the state of relying on someone or something); "independent" means self-reliant, self-sufficient, not needing help.

In the context of Henderson's writings, independence is in need-satisfaction—satisfying one's needs oneself, without relying on another. That health context does not refer to political independence, nor to economic independence, nor to independence in general. Even a very cursory reflection reveals that everyone is dependent on someone or something: on an employer, on traffic lights, on income-tax laws. But when it comes to satisfying basic needs in the area of one's own health, great value is generally put on independence.

Satisfying one's needs on one's own does not imply being isolated from others; being independent in need satisfaction does not mean avoiding fellow human beings. On the contrary, satisfaction of the need to communicate with others presupposes the presence of another person; indeed, for someone to express, for example, his affection or tenderness for another, there must be someone who is willing to receive such attentions. Satisfying the fundamental requirement of working in such a way that there is a sense of accomplishment involves someone who will benefit from the effort; professors require students, producers of goods must have consumers, and providers of services, clients. The "work" of the small child in discovering his world (for example, removing all the pots and pans from the cupboard) not only gives him an enormous sense of accomplishment but also assures him of the almost constant admiration (or, at least, attention) of parent or babysitter.

In everyday conversation, "independence" may have other meanings. The expressions, "she has a much too independent character" and "he'll never manage to become independent" are not necessarily spoken in a health context and probably do not refer to independence in need satisfaction. In the professional context of independence nursing, independence is used in the sense of satisfying one's needs without the help of another.

The importance of respecting the bio-physiological and the psycho-socio-cultural dimensions of fundamental needs when identifying specific needs has already been noted. The same attention is required when considering independence. The newborn infant has, for his stage of development, an independence that differs markedly from that of an adult; parents are justly astonished as they contemplate the extreme independence of their offspring. In his remarkable spontaneity, the baby manages to satisfy his needs at the very moment they make themselves known: he has no inhibitions about communicating his wishes loudly and eloquently, he insists on feedings according to his own private schedule, he goes to sleep and eliminates his body wastes without the slightest concern for company. For his early developmental stage, the baby is very independent in the satisfaction of his needs. Even new parents who refer to their baby as "dependent" on them have to recognize that they are the ones who are dependent on the child.

Independence varies according to other stages also. During pregnancy, a woman is independent in need satisfaction, but differently than at other stages of her life. The elderly person has his own independence, quite different from that he knew at an earlier period. The diabetic may consider himself "dependent" on insulin but be entirely independent in the satisfaction of his needs. The paraplegic may say that he is "dependent" on his wheelchair; he has, however, learned or relearned to satisfy his needs without the help of another. Indeed, he satisfies some of his needs by means of his wheelchair. The independence of the paraplegic is not that of some of his friends, but it is *his* independence. Because specific needs change at different periods of the life span, their satisfaction signifies a different independence.

It is true that some people never know independence in the satisfaction of certain needs; they have, from birth, been forced to depend on someone's help. Others, victims of accident or debilitating illness, never return to their former independence in need satisfaction. The social mandate of the nurse obliges her to maintain the independence that the client has, and to help him to recover the independence that has been lost. When the latter is not possible, the nurse continues her interventions so that the client's needs will be satisfied.

In independence nursing, the client is not qualified as "dependent". He is not dependent as a person, but in relation to the satisfaction of one or more specific needs. For example, if a client cannot satisfy, on his own, his specific need to get up and walk to the armchair in his room twice a day, it is not that he is a dependent person. It is, rather, that he has a dependency problem (he is dependent) for the satisfaction of that particular need, related to, for example, insufficient muscular strength in his left leg. As for some other needs, especially those that are most important in his own eyes, he may be independent.

To continue the example, let us suppose that the nurse's strategy to reinforce his muscular strength is effective and the client does indeed walk to the chair twice a day. His specific need is satisfied—but not independently. As long as he cannot satisfy the need on his own, he has a dependency problem. The nurse therefore continues her intervention; her short-term goal is need satisfaction. However, her middle- or long-term goal is the client's independence in satisfying the need; continuing her complementing-supplementing too long will promote dependence rather than independence. The decision to withdraw her intervention at the appropriate time obviously requires that the nurse have an adequate grounding in the social and biological sciences.

In summary, the goal of the nurse's professional activities is client independence in need satisfaction. A nursing problem is therefore a dependency problem, related to an insufficiency of strength, will, or knowledge. The three sources of difficulty are discussed in the following chapter.

chapter 9

dependency problems

In Virginia Henderson's way of looking at nursing, one cannot but appreciate the clarity of the fourth major unit: the source of difficulty, or the probable origin of the client's health problem that is known as a nursing problem, one that demands the intervention of the health professional known as "nurse". According to Henderson (1966), a health problem, for which one summons a nurse, is a dependency in need-satisfaction; the source of that dependency problem is a lack of strength, will, or knowledge (chapter 3).

Spelling out the source of a dependency problem makes clear the nurse's particular jurisdiction and establishes the boundaries of her special expertise. Rather than attempt to be all things to all people, the nurse recognizes the limits of her service to society; she acknowledges the expertise of other health professionals with whom she is interdependent. That very interdependence presupposes, however, that nursing, as a health profession, has moved from dependency to autonomy; only then can nursing be maturely interdependent (Ford, 1974).

Not all of the client's problems can be handled by the nurse. The client who cannot satisfy his need to eat and drink, because of a lack of money, will require the intervention of someone other than a nurse, because the latter's direct intervention is limited to supplying strength, will, or knowledge. The nurse, of course, provides the client with information about other resource people and may even plead the client's case before the appropriate authorities. And she continues her direct interventions for other unsatisfied needs.

Certain client needs may remain unsatisfied because of a lack of housing or a lack of adequate heating. The nurse does not hesitate to alert those who can intervene directly on those living conditions; she may have to exert considerable pressure on the appropriate authorities so as to obtain services for the client. Acknowledging the limits of her own professional service allows the nurse to call upon other services.

The nurse who practises independence nursing is prepared to solve dependency problems in need satisfaction that are related to an insufficiency of strength, will, or knowledge. The lack (or deficit) will rarely be total. Even with an extremely ill or handicapped person, it is difficult to imagine a total absence of strength, will, and knowledge. It would seem that while there is life, there is a modicum of strength and of will—and perhaps even knowledge. According to Henderson (1966), the nurse completes, increases, or adds to, that which already exists; she seeks to reinforce the already present will, to replace erroneous information with more factual knowledge, and to substitute for the visual strength of the patient whose eyes are temporarily bandaged. It is, therefore, nearly always a case of relative lack or of partial insufficiency. Henderson's conception of the client clearly endows him with his own resources in the way of strength, will, and knowledge. When those resources require complementing and supplementing, the health worker who is prepared to do so, and in such a way that independence in need satisfaction is recovered, is called a *nurse*.

A client's lack of strength is often due to a health problem requiring medical or surgical intervention. Before, during and after that intervention, be it removal of a tumour, reduction of a fracture, or treatment of an infection, the nurse supplements the client's strength so that all his specific needs are satisfied. It is today's satisfaction of needs that allows for a return to independence in their satisfaction at a later date; if certain needs remain unsatisfied, there is little chance that the client will recover his independence related to those needs or indeed to all his needs. The complementarity between health professions is often observed; the physician, because of his particular skills, contributes to the effectiveness of nursing care and the nurse, because of her particular skills, contributes to the effectiveness of medical care. The combined efforts of all members of the interdisciplinary team are necessary for the health and well-being of the beneficiaries of the health care services.

When insufficient strength (muscular, intellectual, cerebral, visual, or other) is the origin of a dependency problem, the client *cannot* satisfy a specific need independently. When a dependency problem is related to a lack of knowledge, the client does *not know* how to satisfy his need and when the source of difficulty is not enough will, he does *not want* to undertake the necessary activity. The statement "does not want to ..." must be qualified; there are three possibilities: the client wants to, but does not want to enough; he wants to and at the same time does not want to; he wants to, but does not dare.

Numerous examples of motivational ambiguity can be found in the general population. One individual may want to lose weight, but does not want to enough to persevere in his efforts. Another is motivated to learn about how to stop smoking but, at the same time, does not want to know any more about the subject. Yet another wants to relax more and work less but does not dare.

Identifying a lack of will, in relation to the non-satisfaction of a need, is not to be interpreted as "blaming" the client. There is no more reproach associated with a lack of motivation than with a lack of strength or knowledge. Everyday expressions such as "he has no will-power" and "he has no motivation" are not part of independence nursing. The nurse does not see "lack of will" as a deliberate refusal by the client; the latter is not lacking motivation because he chooses to have his will-power desert him. It may well be that he *cannot* motivate himself and the underlying factors may be complex and deep-seated and necessitate the long-term intervention of another professional.

Nursing strategies for helping a client motivate or re-motivate himself are not yet well developed. Nursing research in this area, as well as in the areas of supplementing strength and knowledge, may one day provide clinicians with the information that is necessary for their practice of independence nursing.

In the preceding chapter it was pointed out that the client is not qualified as "dependent"; the case is, rather, that in connection with the satisfaction of a specific need, he has a dependency problem. In the same way, the nurse avoids referring to a patient as "lacking knowledge". (Who among us does not lack knowledge about something?) The professional nurse states that the patient does not satisfy a particular need on his own because of insufficient knowledge of how to do so. In other words, the client has a dependency problem related to a lack of knowledge in that area. With regard to another specific need, the client does not have the necessary strength to satisfy it by himself; it is not that the client, in general, lacks strength. When there is a question of insufficient will, it is not that the client, as a person, lacks will-power, but that, related to an unsatisfied specific need, the client does not have the necessary will to satisfy it independently. Anyone interested in the client's care plan, from the client himself to the other members of the interdisciplinary team, must recognize that, by the word "will", the nurse means motivation, volition, psychic energy, and force of will.

The source of a given dependency problem may be an insufficiency of one, or two, or all three resources. A lack of strength is often accompanied by a lack of motivation; insufficient knowledge can coexist with a lack of will. Conversely, without sufficient will, the client's strength and knowledge may be less available to him for the satisfaction of his needs.

A dependency problem cannot be recognized until a specific need has been identified. Before a need is identified, it is quite impossible to see whether it is satisfied independently or not, and if not, why not? The entire second step of the systematic method depends, of course, on the first step: data collection of the bio-physiological and psycho-socio-cultural dimensions of the fundamental need. For each fundamental requirement, several specific needs may be identified, some of which will be satisfied independently, others not. It is therefore impossible, in a clinical situation, to decide that "a fundamental need is satisfied".

For an elderly man who lives alone, a too-hasty conclusion could be drawn, for example, about his fundamental need to avoid dangers. Because he is scrupulously careful about his medications and because he avoids certain foods to which he is allergic, one might be tempted to say that "his fundamental need is satisfied". Yet other "dangers" may exist: loneliness, isolation, tea-and-toast syndrome; until those specific needs have been identified, one cannot say whether or not he is independent in their satisfaction. In the same way, it cannot be assumed that another client's fundamental need to communicate is satisfied because he expresses himself easily and willingly; his fundamental need may be, on the contrary, largely unsatisfied because of other unsatisfied specific needs: making peace with an estranged son or daughter, confiding something important to someone important, sharing with family members a special joy or sadness. A nurse is not expected to work miracles to see that "nothing important gets left unsaid"; she is, however, expected to consider the client's wholeness, and that means identifying his specific needs. Because that identifying must be done together with the client, it contributes to the latter's awareness and may already be a step toward need satisfaction.

In the same line of thought, one cannot assume that the fundamental need to eat and drink is satisfied until the various specific needs proceeding from its bio-physiological and psycho-socio-cultural aspects have been identified.

If the three deficits, lack of strength, will and knowledge, can exist simultaneously for any given need, it is nevertheless important, when only one of them is the source of difficulty, to identify correctly which one is related to the dependency. It is surely a waste of the nurse's time to busy herself doing "patient teaching", when that patient is not lacking information about how to satisfy his need. When the nurse does undertake to increase the client's knowledge, it goes without saying that she will consider timing, teaching methods and appropriate content.

In the same way, a lack of strength must not be confused with a lack of motivation. Reinforcing the muscular strength of the client's arm will not succeed if the origin of the non-satisfaction of the need is really a matter of insufficient motivation. On the other hand, wrongly identifying a lack of will, when the real culprit is a lack of strength (or of knowledge), is not likely to help a client satisfy his needs or recuperate his independence in satisfying them.   Such a mistake will not do anything for nursing's credibility, nor will it increase the client's confidence in his nurse.

The mistake is certainly not as serious as a medication error, for the latter may have immediate and disastrous consequences. The justifiably strict rules that govern the administration of narcotics or other chemicals have no counterpart for guiding the nurse in the identification of the source of a dependency problem. Research in independence nursing may one day provide the required knowledge for not only easier identification of the source of non-satisfaction of needs but also for more effective complementing-supplementing strategies.

The challenge is equally great for both researchers and practitioners. The modes of intervention (increase, replace, etc.) are simple but abstract terms.   Reducing them to empirical indices, that is, translating them into more concrete terms, calls upon every nurse's creativity, initiative and intuition as well as a wealth of scientific knowledge.

When there is no dependency problem in need satisfaction, no deficit has to be identified. The nurse works to prevent dependency problems by maintaining client independence. Potential problems may, however, be identified and means taken to prevent them. Prevention always requires planning, whether the clientele consists of school children, pregnant women, the soon-to-retire or any other target group, or indeed any individual. If the client's current needs are satisfied, the nurse's experience may incite her to predict future needs, which, without sufficient planning, may be more difficult to satisfy.

The prediction and prevention of potential problems does not mean inventing future problems, as though the nurse feared that her complementary-supplementary role might became socially insignificant. In the same way that specific needs must be real and realistic, so also dependency problems in need satisfaction must be real and realistic.   Both are identified with the active participation of the client, and the latter is the one who has the last word. Henderson (1988) insists that, for any given client, the nurse must make herself dispensable as quickly as possible. The nurse who sees to it that she remains indispensable is not promoting client independence.

Alderman (1980) discusses the client's self-responsibility for health and explores the reasons why some people do not accept that responsibility; same "can" not, others "will" not. Those who can, have the necessary strength, ability, or skill; when they cannot, it is often because they lack knowledge of what to do and how to do it. As for those who "will" not, they are lacking motivation, intention, effort. Alderman points out that if motivation or will is present, the person is likely to overcome a lack of ability (knowledge, skill). The same author underlines the importance for health professionals to identify correctly the causal factor.

Alderman's (1980) discussion on self-responsibility calls to mind Henderson's early writings. More than thirty years ago (Harmer & Henderson, 1955), she conceptualized nursing's contribution to health: the complementing-supplementing of the client's strength, will, and knowledge so that his independence in need satisfaction would be maintained and restored.

chapter 10

relating other concepts to independence nursing

The purpose of this chapter is to discuss the link between various concepts and Henderson's conceptual model for nursing. Because a conceptual model is sometimes seen as excluding all except its own concepts, the point must be made.

One of the most frequently heard arguments against nursing models is that they limit nurses to a narrow or restricted viewpoint, *i.e.*, a precise conceptual model for nursing is seen as limiting, confining, and prohibiting the study of new and interesting scientific discoveries. Educators and practitioners refuse, with good reason, to be stifled by artificially impenetrable boundaries.

While it is true that a conceptual model delineates the scope of nursing in that the ideal and limited goal is defined and the role of the nurse is circumscribed, nevertheless the limits set are in no way confining and the boundaries are not impervious. On the contrary, a frame of reference that specifies how nursing views the client, and how nursing helps him, places on nurses the heavy obligation of keeping abreast of any scientific progress that concerns health. The almost constant addition to existing knowledge in the biological and human sciences can be useful to nurses precisely because they have a framework to which the new information can be attached and integrated with already acquired scientific knowledge. A conceptual model is therefore a liberating force; it incites nurses to be receptive to any new knowledge that will help them achieve their professional goal.

A concept is formed and developed in the mind following an experience or the acquisition of knowledge. The word or symbol used to name the concept varies among individuals. The mental image of the unpleasant physical feeling caused by a twisted ankle or a smashed thumb is probably the same for everyone; the symbol used to verbalize the sensation differs with each language: pain, "schmerz", "dor", "douleur."

The inverse is also true, as the same word does not necessarily provoke the same mental image for everyone. Sunday dinner, for example, is doubtless not quite the same for a Canadian family as for a Mexican one. Even within the same profession words are often deceptive. The writer recalls a hospital setting where the nursing assessment was known as the nursing history. During an orientation period for newly engaged nurses, the programme announced a talk on the subject "nursing history". The new staff members attended reluctantly, believing they were about to hear a speech on the history of nursing.*

We have already seen that a conceptual model is a mental image, an invention of the mind, a conception, a way of conceptualizing reality. The mental image of a profession is a very complex concept which, in its turn, includes other concepts such as the goal of the profession and the role of the professional. Virginia Henderson has made explicit her way of conceptualizing nursing; the result is a very complex concept within which are others such as need, independence, etc.

It may seem pretentious to speak of teaching a concept. Since it forms and develops in the mind of the student, a concept can hardly be taught. The facts and details that go toward the formation of the concept can, however, be taught; in schools of nursing as well as in in-service programmes, the teacher's responsibility is to provide the learner with opportunities to acquire facts and experience new things that will permit the student to form concepts in harmony with reality. For example, the educator will choose clinical experiences, films, books and discussions that will help the student develop, in his mind, a concept of circulatory shock that corresponds to that physiopathologic reality.

---

* Questioned on what "medical history" meant to them, the same nurses replied that it was the information the doctor needed to obtain from the patient in order to help him.

Our study of the fundamental needs reveals that each one has bio-physiological and psycho-socio-cultural aspects. The client of nursing is a human being; it follows, therefore, that whatever influences his fundamental needs is of interest to the nurse. Far from narrowing her visual field, the conceptual model stimulates the nurse continually to add to her knowledge so as to be better prepared to pursue her particular goal. New concepts arising from biochemistry, nuclear physics, psychology or medicine, to name but a few disciplines, are useful to the nurse inasmuch as they influence the client's independence in need satisfaction.

Some examples of concepts of particular interest to nurses now follow. No attempt is made to explain them, nor is the list in any way complete. The examples are mentioned in the hope of demonstrating that the adoption of a conceptual model is entirely compatible with the use of many diverse concepts such as the concepts of grief and mourning, pain, body image, sensory deprivation, sensory overload, stress and alternative approaches.

grief and mourning

The psycho-social sciences provide us with a wealth of information about the significance to human beings of suffering a loss. Following an important loss, such as the death of a loved one, the amputation of a limb, or a loss of some body function, a person goes through the steps of grieving and mourning. This highly complex process involves other concepts such as denial and anger. It is more than likely that, during the work of mourning, the client's independence is affected in some way and his individual needs have changed because of the loss. If so, the nurse's intervention must be adapted or modified.

It is evident that a woman who has recently undergone a mastectomy has very personal needs with regard to moving, eliminating, and communicating her feelings, to name only three of her basic needs. Depending on the meaning she herself gives to the amputation of her breast, she works through, in her own way and at her own rhythm, the various stages of mourning her loss. If the nurse has some knowledge of the concept of mourning, she will use that knowledge in helping the patient express her feelings and learn to care for herself. In her inter-personal relationship, with the client and her family, the nurse will be more attentive and respectful of their feelings and behaviour than if she had no understanding of the complex work of mourning.

Similarly, a man who has suffered a myocardial infarct undoubtedly mourns the loss of his youthful vigour, the para-plegic grieves for the recent loss of movement of his lower limbs, and the mother of a still-born baby mourns the loss of her child. The family of each person also has to work through the loss and grief. To the extent that the work of mourning affects need satisfaction, it is a useful, if not indispensable, concept for the nurse.

pain

This particularly complex concept, with its neuro-physio-logical, psychological, and socio-cultural ramifications, may affect the client's independence in the satisfaction of *all* his needs. The pain suffered by the patient with trigeminal neuralgia, for example, seriously reduces his ability to eat and to care for his teeth. The pain of the arthritic may prevent him from moving about, seeking diversion or doing useful work at will. Even the anticipation of pain, as before a diagnostic test, may prevent the patient from requesting the information he wants about the test. The more the nurse knows about pain in all its many dimensions, the more helpful she will be to the client whose independence is modified because of his suffering.

body image

The biological and social sciences acquaint us with the long and extremely complex development, in every human being, of his own body image. A patient's physical self-concept may be disturbed by a health problem; the disturbance, in turn, may affect the patient's independence in need satisfaction. The nurse must have some knowledge of body image and use the concept in her nursing care.

It is not surprising to find that a person with a permanent colostomy has suffered considerable disturbance of his body image. Added to his immediate personal needs (*e.g.*, the areas of cleanliness, elimination, eating and drinking, etc.) are needs generated not by the surgery itself but by the alteration of his body image or physical self-concept. For example, the patient may be anxious about resuming his sexual relations (need to communicate) and pessimistic about going to the theatre (need for diversion) and participating in long business meetings (need to do useful work). The nurse with some knowledge of the results of an altered body image and of the sub-concepts of denial, fear of rejection, and the like, will understand why the patient refuses to look at his colostomy during the initial post-operative care. She will not immediately launch into a long explanation of the approved technique that the patient must learn in order to care for himself and, despite his need to learn the care of his colostomy, she will begin by helping him to accept the reality of his new situation and to overcome his repugnance toward his artificial anus.

Understanding the concept of body image and its various implications gives the nurse a special awareness of the obese person, the hemiplegic, the disfigured accident victim, the adolescent humiliated by his acne, and so forth. Because she is sensitive to the fact that even a threat to body image may modify individual needs, she will understand the distress of a client faced with a treatment or examination that requires the penetration of a body cavity by a diagnostic instrument and she will then adjust her explanations to the needs of the client. In the same line of thinking, the nurse is sensitive to the child's fear of a rectal thermometer. It appears that even an oral thermometer can be threatening for a child if the nurse who approaches him says "I am going to TAKE your temperature." Children who are accustomed to having their temperature TAKEN are of course not threatened; body image is not always disturbed, but when it is, the nurse owes it to herself and to her patient to recognize the phenomenon.

sensory deprivation

It seems that the human being is not indifferent to the reduction or the absence of the sensory stimulation to which he has become accustomed. When a client of the health services suffers that type of deprivation, it cannot but influence the satisfaction of his needs and, therefore, the nurse's interventions.

Isolation technique deprives a patient, at least in part, of a variety of stimulation, *e.g.*, *tactile* (the personnel wears gloves), *visual* (visitors and personnel wear masks and gowns), *gustatory* (meals are served on cardboard dishes), and perhaps *auditory* and *olfactive* (reduced contact with the world at large). Being aware of the implications of sensory deprivation for her patient, the nurse will be attentive to certain specific needs if they arise. The nurse may help the client communicate his feelings of isolation, avoid the psychological dangers of sensory monotony, and maintain certain physical exercises.

The concept of sensory deprivation, still within Henderson's framework, is useful in the care of the dying and of their families. The nurse who flees the client in his last hours deprives him and his family of important sensory stimulation (tactile and auditory). Similarly, she contributes to the sensory deprivation of the unconscious client when she abandons all efforts at verbal communication.

The social isolation of the chronically ill and the aged are other aspects of sensory deprivation that affect the satisfaction of specific needs and consequently the nurse's interventions.

sensory overload

A client also suffers from the opposite of sensory deprivation: sensory overload. Here again, specific needs may be greatly changed. The nurse will be particularly attentive to an increase in confronting stimuli in coronary care and intensive care units. Patients in these areas may be constantly assaulted by noise as well as by visual (lights on day and night) and tactile (tubes, instruments, machines) stimulation. Such a situation presents a challenge to the nurse who seeks to help the patient satisfy his particular needs for rest and sleep.

The client at home, or in the quieter areas of the hospital, may sometimes suffer from an excess of visitors, noise, or pain. During the period of sensory overload, his individual needs are considerably modified.

stress

Everyone, including health professionals, lives daily with a certain stress. If health problems are often the result of too much stress, they are also the frequent cause of increased stress. A change in emotional state, the waiting period before being admitted to hospital and the pronouncement of a diagnosis, are all examples of sources of stress that the nurse must recognize, since they will have their impact on her client's independence in satisfying his needs.

alternative approaches

Under the loose heading of "alternative treatment modalities" are found therapeutic touch, massage, visualization, and others. They are used in independence nursing as complementing-supplementing interventions. Specific needs in the areas of communicating and learning, to name only two examples, sometimes respond to "alternative approaches"; the latter must therefore be part of the nurse's repertoire.

An alternative approach does not become a conceptual base for nursing. An intervention is chosen only after duly collecting data, identifying specific needs and their source of non-satisfaction.

summary

Any other concept that touches the client's wholeness and his independence in need satisfaction should be understood by nurses: growth and development, poverty, role satisfaction, loneliness, reminiscence, reality orientation, etc. Knowledge of such concepts may influence one or more of the steps of the systematic process. The greater the nurse's knowledge of human nature, the better prepared she is to make astute observations, identify subtle needs, recognize dependency problems and choose effective complementary-supplementary interventions.

Each one of the concepts discussed is, in itself, an intellectually stimulating idea, already sufficient reason to learn about it. If as well, the concept helps us to provide better nursing care because it contributes to our understanding of the client, it becomes doubly interesting. As knowledge continues to multiply in all disciplines, the nurse, more than ever before, has reason to have a specific conceptual framework that will help her put to good use new and developing knowledge. The helping relationship is woven of respect and understanding—attitudes that are developed, at least partly, from the knowledge of a wide range of concepts.

chapter 11

independence nursing and community health

Conceptual models for nursing all have, as the second major unit, a term for conceptualizing "person" as the client of nursing. The term does not offer a philosophical conception of "person" nor of person as parent, friend or spouse; what it offers is a conception of person-as-client of nursing. The authors of the extant models for nursing indicate that the client may be an individual, a family, or a group, yet many nurses consider that the descriptive term used is relevant only to a client-individual. Because nurses have long practised in a variety of settings, their client has often been a group or even a community. This chapter will explore the utility of Henderson's model for nursing in a community health setting.

Nurses who are interested in community health rightly consider the hospital as part of the community; a hospitalized patient is still a member of his family and of his community. However, the same nurses often come to feel that health promotion and the prevention of health problems have less importance in the hospital than they do in other care settings. Community nurses want to be recognized as being health oriented (rather than illness oriented) and are justly proud to be members of the interdisciplinary health team. All members of that team are faced with a bewildering variety of definitions of "health".

The very complexity of that most precious commodity makes health difficult to define, that is, to set forth its essence, to declare its exact meaning and scope. There is some agreement that health is more than the absence of illness, but consensus does not go much further.

For some, health is a process, for others, a dynamic state. Bruhn *et al.* (1977) and Dunn (1959) make a distinction between health and wellness, the latter going beyond mere health. Wu (1973), however, sees health and wellness as synonymous. Crawford (1977) questions the "right" to health and health care.

More than forty definitions of health provided by philosophers, nurses, physicians and others have been analyzed by Keller (1981), using various sub-concepts such as harmony, heredity, and environment; among the sub-concepts, biophysiology ranked highest in the definitions, holism, lowest.

Newman (1986) presents a synthesized view of health, one that incorporates disease as a meaningful aspect of health; "health includes disease and disease includes health" (p. 9).

Many health professionals make up the interdisciplinary team, and all are committed to preserving and promoting health; no one alone is sufficient to the task. "It is unlikely that nursing alone has been or will be given the responsibility of safeguarding health" (Johnson, 1978, p. 6). Regardless of its preferred definition of health, each profession must have a clear and explicit conception of its particular contribution *to* health.

Nursing's singular contribution to health is, according to Henderson (1966), the maintaining and restoring of client independence in need satisfaction. This discipline model does not define health; it is a conception of nursing. If any one discipline's contribution *to* health were, at the same time, its definition *of* health, then that discipline would indeed see itself as sufficient to the task of promoting health.

A nurse is educated to offer a particular service to society; it is not logical for her to change her conception of that service according to her work setting any more than it would be reasonable for her to change her frame of reference according to the client's medical diagnosis. The shifting of the conceptual base is, of course, not always acknowledged. It is interesting to note that when a psychologist is working with a person who has a cardiac problem, the psychologist is not heard to say that he or she is "doing cardiac psychology"; a dietician who works with post-partum patients does not refer to obstetrical dietetics any more than a social worker might refer to diabetic social work.

Yet nurses are still known to state that they are "doing psychiatric nursing", or "orthopedic nursing" or "neurological nursing".

Qualifying the word "nursing" with a medical specialty reveals that the nurse adopts, in large part, the frame of reference of, for example, the cardiologist or the psychiatrist. When that nurse adopts a distinct nursing perspective, she is "doing independence nursing" (or "adaptation nursing"), whatever her client's medical diagnosis and whatever her work setting. She will strive to promote client independence (or client adaptation) in a hospital setting as much as she will in the community.

It is important to reflect on the influence that a nurse's conceptual base can exert on her practice. A nurse sometimes leaves the hospital setting for a community one, in order to remove herself from the "medically oriented" hospital; she eagerly becomes a school nurse, an industrial nurse or a community health centre nurse, so that she will not only work in a health-oriented setting but so that she will also be autonomous. Unless she has a distinct nursing perspective, she will, consciously or otherwise, borrow another's conceptual base; replacing the medical perspective with an epidemiological or sociological perspective, to name only two possibilities, will only underline her *lack* of professional autonomy. Even if she has no medical orders to carry out, even if she no longer consults a physician, she may still have a medical perspective; being alone does not necessarily confer autonomy.

As stated in chapter 9, interdependence among the members of the health team is possible only when each member-discipline is sure of its professional identity. The following figure represents the interdependence and the independence of various health disciplines. The shaded areas show the inevitable overlapping; many tasks can be carried out by one or the other. However, each discipline has a particular contribution to health and that contribution justifies its presence on the team.

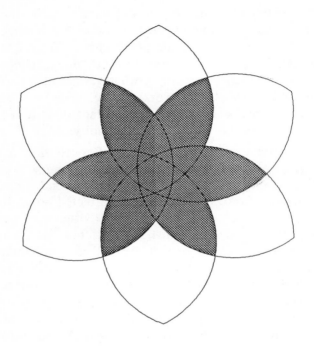

Interdisciplinary Health Team

The community nurse who is committed to independence nursing will strive to maintain independence in need satisfaction with an individual, with a family, or with a group. Each type of client has fourteen fundamental needs, but the specific needs that derive from the fundamental ones differ greatly, depending on the client. For each type of client, the nurse must have abundant knowledge.

When the client is a group of elderly people, the nurse must have knowledge of group dynamics and about aging; she must also have a clear idea of her social role as a nurse. When the client is a group of diabetic teenagers, the nurse must have knowledge of groups, of diabetes and of adolescence; she must also have an explicit conception of how she, as a nurse, can help them. When the client is a family, the nurse must have knowledge of family structure and functioning; she must also be clear about what constitutes her particular professional competence. Just as the nurse who identifies the specific needs of the woman who is pregnant, or of the man who has just suffered a myocardial infarct, must have knowledge about pregnancy and about cardiology, so also, the nurse who recognizes the specific needs of a family must have knowledge about that complex entity. In each situation, the bio-physiological and the psycho-socio-cultural dimensions of each fundamental need give rise to a variety of specific needs. And in each situation, the nurse must be aware of her professional goal, of her social role, and of all the other components of her distinct nursing perspective.

Nursing intervention with a family is vastly different from nursing intervention with an individual (Latourelle, 1985; Wright & Leahey, 1984). Specializing in family nursing requires extensive graduate preparation.

In the context of independence nursing, the nurse's goal is to maintain and restore family independence in need satisfaction. Data collection is done in an encounter with all family members; the family participates in identifying its specific needs and in determining their priority. Within a given family, priorities will of course change from one time period to another; again, Maslow's hierarchy may prove helpful in establishing priority. Family members will decide, together with the nurse, on strategies to complement their strength, will, or knowledge.

An assessment tool to be used with a client-family will be very different from that used with a client-individual. What follows is a non-exhaustive list of items to be considered in the construction of an assessment tool to be used with families.

1. Eat and drink adequately

Family traditions; importance given to food and to family togetherness at meal-time; rules for table manners; tolerance for individual tastes and preferences; attitudes toward breast-feeding; division of labour in meal preparation.

2. Breathe normally

Ratio of number of rooms to number of family members; ventilation; humidity of the dwelling; number of smokers; quality of air in the neighbourhood.

3. Eliminate body wastes

Ratio of toilets, bathrooms to number of family members; sewage system in the area; family rules regarding individual privacy; attitudes toward toilet training.

4. Move and maintain desirable postures

Freedom of movement in the dwelling (stairs, arrangement of rooms and furniture); family outings (outside stairs, family car, holidays, recreation); flexibility of "reserved" places (chairs, place at table); special requirements of some family members.

5. Sleep and rest

Ratio of bedrooms to number of family members; neighbour-hood noise; importance given to rest and sleep; respect for privacy; tolerance of individual schedules, preferences.

6. Dress and undress

Flexibility-rigidity of family rules and standards; social desirability; importance of individual preferences (teenager, aged member); division of responsibility (care of clothing, financial).

7. Maintain body temperature

Heating and ventilation of dwelling; individual tolerance (baby, aging member); respect for individual preferences.

8. Keep the body clean

Ratio of bathrooms to number of family members; family rules (personal hygiene, household cleanliness); division of cleaning tasks; rules about table manners; toilet training.

9. Avoid dangers and avoid injuring others

Threats to the family (alcohol, drugs, pregnancy, eviction, suicide); incomplete grieving; family member leaving home; breakdown of communications; consequences of illness of a family member.

10. Communicate with others in expressing emotions, needs, fears, or opinions

Taboo subjects; role of members in family interactions; rules about expressing emotions, pleasant and unpleasant; family interaction; privacy of parents and siblings; sexual education of children; family interaction with community, with health services, with extended family; importance given to clarity in communication.

11. Worship according to one's faith

Spiritual or religious practices as a family; importance given to spirituality; flexibility-rigidity of family rules; respect for individual practices; influence of religion on diet, play, use of health services.

12. Work in such a way that there is a sense of accomplishment

Family obligations regarding the community, the extended family; political and social commitments; roles of family members (child, parent, spouse); respect for different social roles (student, wage-earner, retired worker, homemaker); division of labour within the family; importance given to achievements; family solidarity.

13. Play or participate in various forms of recreation

Relaxation as a family (weekends, holidays, outings); family traditions (special days, family reunions); rules regarding television, choice of friends, inviting people in; curfew rules; respect for individual preferences; importance given to recreation.

14. Learn, discover ...

Value put on studying, learning; use of health and other community services; interest in satisfaction of other needs (communicating, playing); ways of coping with situational crises (illness, death, loss of work); ways of treating conflict between members.

Bio-physiological dimensions of each need vary from family to family and within a family from time to time. The parents may be young or elderly; the family may include young children or an aging grandparent. A pregnancy, an illness, a handicapped member, or a parent who carries a genetic defect are examples of bio-physiological factors that influence family dynamics.

The psycho-socio-cultural dimensions of each need are equally important. One family may be preoccupied by its reputation in the community, by the way it is perceived by others; another may consider itself as an influential leader. The family experiencing death, separation, divorce, loss of work, retirement, abortion, or illness has different specific needs from the one experiencing the happy arrival of a new baby, a wedding, scholastic success, or professional achievement. The socio-cultural context may be permissive or restrictive; the linguistic and religious background, the economic and political climate may influence the family needs to eat and to dress quite as much as their needs to communicate, to play, and to work in such a way that there is a sense of accomplishment.

The fact that the nurse is working with the family-as-client does not prevent her from also having one or more members of the family as client-individuals. The needs of the family, as a family, are not the same as the individual member's needs but, because of family interaction, what touches one family member touches all other members and touches the family as an entity. For example, certain specific needs of a sick member will alter a family need; a particular family need will, in turn, modify the specific needs of the sick member.

The nurse whose client is a family puts to good use her skills in establishing, maintaining and terminating an interpersonal relationship that the family will consider a helping one. The quality of the client-nurse relationship will determine the effectiveness of the nursing intervention, whether the client is a family or an individual. Given the complexity of family interaction, the judicious and effective complementing of family motivation and family knowledge could conceivably exert an influence on family health for generations to come.

Other members of the interdisciplinary health team may also have occasion to intervene with the family. Each one does so according to his specific expertise, each one according to his particular professional goal.

Independence nursing also permits the community nurse to develop programmes for pre-retirement groups, pregnant women, factory workers or any other type of clientele. Again, the needs of the group, as a group, will not be the same as those of the individual members. When the programme is an interdisciplinary one, the nurse, sure of her professional identity and confident about the value of her particular contribution to society's health, will rejoice in the interdependence of the health team members.

As any other professional nurse, the one who chooses to work in a community health setting wants to practise her own profession; her contribution to health is not to help another health worker practise his or her profession. To be autonomous, the nurse must have a conceptual frame of reference that is sufficiently clear and explicit as to orient her observations and her actions and to permit her to assert herself as a full-fledged member of the health team. It would seem that independence nursing is compatible not only with professional autonomy but also with community health.

chapter 12

independence nursing and nursing diagnosis

The expression "nursing diagnosis" has been part of nursing terminology for some time and has become a familiar and popular concept for practitioners, researchers and educators. Not everyone, however, understands the expression in the same way. As with any concept, "nursing diagnosis" can be a useful one for nursing or it can, on the contrary, be abused to the point of becoming a disservice to the profession.

England (1989) presents various definitions of nursing diagnosis, including the one accepted by the North American Nursing Diagnosis Association: "nursing diagnoses are responses to actual or potential health problems that nurses by virtue of their education and experience are able, licensed, and legally responsible and accountable to treat" (p. 349).

For some nurses (Anderson & Briggs, 1988; Kritek, 1979), a diagnostic statement is the result of nursing assessment; it is the second step of the systematic method known as the "nursing process". Carpenito (1983), on the other hand, claims that nursing diagnosis will define nursing, classify nursing's domain and differentiate nursing from medicine*; she seems to see nursing diagnosis as an alternative to a conceptual model. Fawcett (1986) describes nursing diagnosis as middle-range descriptive naming theory.

Nurse educators have been heard to state that their university programme is "based on" nursing diagnosis; it would seem that

---

* As an example of a clinical medical problem, Carpenito (p. 15) gives "Levin tube" and, as an example of the corresponding clinical nursing problem, "potential aspiration".

those educators give to nursing diagnosis the status of a conceptual base for a programme in nursing science.

Numerous formulations and classifications of nursing diagnoses have been published. In a study to determine their diagnostic content validity, Levin *et al.* (1989) quote the six most frequently used diagnoses (p. 43):

- Comfort, Alteration in: Pain
- Mobility, Impaired Physical
- Skin Integrity, Impairment of: Actual
- Knowledge Deficit (Specify)
- Self-Care Deficit—feeding, bathing, dressing, toileting
- Anxiety.

Levine (1989) is wary of nursing diagnosis language and of the subtle messages it may be sending; as an example, she wonders what a surgeon must think when he reads the following nursing diagnosis for a patient on whom he has performed a colostomy: "Patient has alteration in bowel movement" (p. 5). Probably every reader has personally observed the embarrassing incidents that can occur when lists of nursing diagnoses are provided in a clinical setting accompanied by the obligation for all nurses to write a nursing diagnosis on every patient care plan. Obliging a nurse to choose, from a prepared list of diagnoses, a nursing diagnosis for her client could well be a meaningless requirement unless that nurse has an explicit nursing frame of reference for the entire systematic process.

A medical diagnosis reflects a medical perspective; all medical diagnoses seem to refer to structural (anatomic) or functional (physiological) stress. An economic "diagnosis" reveals an economic way of looking at reality and an architectural "diagnosis" reflects an architectural frame of reference. Each diagnosis follows the important step of data collection; that important step always has a conceptual base.

A nursing diagnosis will, logically, reflect the conceptual model for nursing on which the entire systematic process is based. If Henderson's way of looking at nursing provides the conceptual base of that process, what then would be a nursing diagnosis?

We have seen (chapter 4) that, in independence nursing, the second step of the clinical process is the identification of a specific need, a decision about its satisfaction or non-satisfaction and the related source of dependency. Example: specific need to drink 200 cc of liquid q. 2 h, not satisfied independently owing to a lack of strength to swallow (or to insufficient strength of both hands, to not enough motivation, to a lack of knowledge about the reasons to force fluids, to name only a few possibilities). For each specific need identified, a problem statement, that is, a dependency in need-satisfaction statement, is made:

- (Specific need to) express his fear of the diagnosis, not satisfied independently because of insufficient motivation (he does not *dare*).
- (Specific need to) rest 1-2 h every afternoon, not satisfied independently related to lack of strength to overcame his anxiety (he *can't*).

In this way, multiple problem statements are made for each client. No one problem statement alone constitutes the client's diagnosis; each one is, rather, a mini-diagnosis or a partial diagnosis. Each problem statement reflects the nurse's social mission to maintain or restore client independence in need satisfaction.

The combined work of practitioners, researchers and educators who are committed to independence nursing may one day reveal a grouping, or combining, of several problem statements in a "syndrome". A diagnostic label—signifying that grouping— would then be known. The grouping might be according to fundamental needs, to one or the other of the need's dimensions, or according to the lack (of strength, will, or knowledge).

Nurses who have another conceptual base would couch the problem statements in terms of behavioral equilibrium (Johnson), or of adaptation (Roy), or in some other terms that reflect their conceptual framework, one that gives explicit direction for nursing practice, education, and research.

For the moment, nursing diagnoses such as the six most frequently used that are quoted above must be "translated" if they are to reflect independence nursing. For example, "Mobility, Impaired Physical" could be, for a given client "(specific need to) walk fifteen minutes each day, not satisfied independently owing to insufficient knowledge of how to use crutches". For another client, the same diagnosis, "Mobility, Impaired Physical" would translate into something entirely different.

Carpenito's (1983) claim that nursing diagnosis will define nursing's subject matter and distinguish nursing from medicine will be justified only if nursing diagnoses truly reflect nursing's particular social mission in the health arena. Surely nursing diagnoses must be *based on* an explicit nursing framework rather than *be* the conceptual base. Fawcett (1986) states that nursing diagnosis will "become an integral and meaningful part of nursing science and nursing practice [...] if further development of nursing diagnosis is clearly based on explicit assumptions that are part of a conceptual model of nursing" (p. 397).

This writer is concerned that further development of nursing diagnosis may not be in nursing's best interests. Nursing has long boasted that it considers the whole person; if adequate diagnostic labels were found, it is conceivable that nursing would eventually forsake its holistic viewpoint and fall a prey to the temptation (already recognized elsewhere) of treating the diagnosis, not the person as a whole. Perhaps nursing should resist, as some other helping professions have done, the very notion of "diagnosis". Independence nursing should perhaps continue to consider that some specific needs are satisfied independently by the client, while others are associated with dependency problems and require the complementing-supplementing interventions of a nurse. It may not be worthwhile to seek a diagnostic label that would cover all or many of a client's dependency problems in need satisfaction.

Nursing has no obligation to emulate medicine's success in developing diagnostic labels that are so well known that they are recognized even by people outside the medical profession. If, however, nursing diagnoses are to be further developed, care must be taken that they are truly *nursing* diagnoses.

chapter 13

beyond the conceptual model

As already stated, a conceptual model for a professional discipline provides direction for that discipline's practice, research and education and, of course, for the administration of those three fields of activity. The chosen frame of reference is the conceptual departure point, the conceptual skeleton or framework on which further construction is done and to which advanced developments are attached.

Henderson's conception of what nursing could or should be is sufficiently complete and explicit as to warrant the appellation "conceptual model for nursing". From that conceptual departure point or framework can be considered the development of nursing theory, the advancement of nursing science, and the examination of what has become known, at least to some, as nursing's metaparadigm.

nursing theory

The definitions of the word "theory" that have come from various disciplines have been widely quoted by nurse authors; Roy & Roberts (1981) have combined the elements of several definitions: "A theory is a system of interrelated propositions used to describe, predict, explain, understand, and control a part of the empirical world" (p. 5). Parse (1987) specifies further that a theory "explains, describes, or makes predictions about the phenomena of a discipline" (p. 2).

A nursing theory must therefore be a theory. The word "nursing" will distinguish it from biological theory or from physical or psychological theory. "Phenomena of a discipline" and "part of the empirical world" will be *nursing* phenomena and *nursing's* empirical world. The nurse's conceptual frame of reference will indicate nursing's focus of inquiry, that is, the phenomena that are of particular concern to nursing.

Henderson's frame of reference indicates that the profession's focus of inquiry includes wholeness, need (fundamental and specific), need satisfaction, independence in need satisfaction, complementary-supplementary strategies and others. Nursing theories would therefore be of and about those phenomena. The knowledge generated would be essential for nursing practice; it might well prove useful to other health disciplines also. Knowledge does not ever belong exclusively to the discipline that develops it. When other disciplines make use of it, they are not "borrowing" knowledge; they are merely availing themselves of existing knowledge. Nursing theories may one day be as useful to related disciplines as existing theories, developed in other fields, are today useful to nursing.

The multiple theories that could be developed from Henderson's way of looking at nursing would be of various types. Fawcett (1985) points out that theory may be descriptive and developed by exploratory research; it may be explanatory theory, developed by correlational research or predictive theory, developed by experimental research. Chinn & Jacobs (1983) use such theory classifications as "macro", "midrange", and "micro".

None of the foregoing qualifications, however, will replace the word "nursing". For a theory to be predictive (or descriptive, macro, or any other) theory in nursing, it must be of and about those phenomena that are of particular concern to nursing in the sense that knowledge about them is required for nursing practice. The theory would not be a theory of nursing; it would be, in the case of independence nursing, a theory of independence or a theory of need satisfaction, to name only two possibilities.

Even when multiple theories will have been developed from the conceptual starting point of Henderson's conception of nursing, that same conception will still guide practice, research, and education. The fact that various theories explain and describe the phenomena of interest to nursing does not in any way obviate the importance of continuing to have an explicit way of conceptualizing the discipline. No amount of refinement or "further research" will transform a conceptual model into a theory. A way of looking at an entire profession will not be replaced by, nor changed into, a system of propositions used to explain and predict the phenomena of interest to that same profession.

Several authors (Bush, 1979; Fawcett, 1978; Newman, 1979) support the notion that conceptual models are precursors of theory. Others (Meleis, 1985; Silva, 1986; Stevens, 1979) do not consider important the distinction between the two terms.

Henderson's model for nursing, made up of assumptions, values, and major units (as presented in this book), contains no propositions, validated or otherwise, no hypotheses, confirmed or not. In short, it is not a theory, to be "tested". According to Johnson (1974), "the question of 'truth' plays no part in judging a model for nursing practice, education and research based on the conceptual system" (p. 376). A model is not "right" or "wrong"; it is a way of conceptualizing what nursing could or should be. A model may prove worthless, but not because it is not true. If it proves worthless, it is because it does not meet the criteria for its evaluation.

Johnson (1974) has developed extrinsic criteria for evaluating a conceptual model: social congruence, social significance, and social utility. They signify that social decisions will judge a model by the service that is based on it; clients will respond to such questions as "Is nursing congruent with your expectations?", "Is nursing meaningful, significant to your health?" and many others.

Intrinsic criteria for evaluating a model are clarity, precision and coherency in the assumptions, values and major units.

Henderson's complementary-supplementary model may one day give rise to a system of propositions known as, for example, a theory of complementing motivation in the elderly related to their need to play, or a theory of supplementing knowledge for chemotherapy patients with regard to their need to eat and drink. This would require extensive research, making use of all the extant knowledge that the social and biological sciences have to offer. Just as medicine makes use of knowledge of anatomy and biochemistry to study the problems of preventing, diagnosing, and treating illness, so also nursing will use, for example, knowledge of psychology and physiology to study the problems of preventing, identifying, and alleviating dependency in need satisfaction.

When nurses study phenomena that are also of interest to other disciplines, they will do so from a nursing perspective. For example, pain may be studied from a psychological, anthropological, or medical perspective, thus generating knowledge useful to more than one discipline. If pain were studied from Henderson's frame of reference, it would be because pain is a phenomenon that interferes with need satisfaction and with independence in need satisfaction. The knowledge generated would, conceivably, be useful to more than one health discipline.

The possibilities for the development of nursing theory are numerous and exciting. But the key word is *nursing*. Research done from a borrowed perspective, or from one that is not also the conceptual base for practice and education, or from one that is not clear and explicit, can hardly be expected to develop *nursing* theory. If the researcher's conception of nursing is not one that is also useful for practice and education, the researcher is distancing herself from her discipline; she is not likely, therefore, to develop the knowledge that is necessary for nursing practice. And if nursing research is based on the perspective of another discipline, it is more likely to contribute to the advancement of that other discipline than to the development of nursing.

nursing science

Closely related to nursing theory, nursing science is an advanced development that can be built from Henderson's way of looking at nursing.

Science has been defined as a systematic body of knowledge (Dessler, 1980 in Gruending, 1985), as a consensual informed opinion about the natural world, rather than a body of codified knowledge (Gortner & Schultz, 1988) and as a process of knowing and challenging (Newman, 1983). For Greene (1979), science is both a process (the scientific method) and a body of organized knowledge (rather than intuitive or common knowledge).

According to Johnson (1974), sciences "become differentiated from one another on the basis of what is studied and the perspective used to raise questions, make observations and interpret evidence" (p. 373). The same author insists that "... it is the distinctive perspective of each science which most clearly discriminates it from others" (p. 373).

"Nursing" then, is once more the key word in differentiating nursing science from others. Nursing science will be a systematic body of *nursing* knowledge, a process of knowing and challenging in *nursing*.

What would constitute nursing knowledge? A nurse who has a bio-medical vision of nursing will consider bio-medical knowledge as nursing knowledge. If her conception of nursing is borrowed from epidemiology, then epidemiological knowledge will be, for her, nursing knowledge. Qualifying knowledge as bio-chemical, for example, does not mean it is not used by other disciplines; it only means that bio-chemistry, in pursuing its focus of scientific inquiry, has developed the knowledge.

A nurse who has adopted Henderson's vision of nursing will consider, as nursing knowledge, that which is developed for maintaining and restoring client independence in need satisfaction. Nursing knowledge will be about wholeness, independence, etc. Nursing science will be the process of knowing and challenging with regard to needs, need satisfaction, etc.

Of itself, a conceptual model for nursing does not constitute nursing knowledge. It is not a definition of nursing. It cannot be considered a knowledge base for nursing. A conceptual model is merely a way of conceptualizing what nursing could or should be; as such, it indicates the kind of knowledge that must be sought.

Little is known, at the moment, about complementing client strength, will, and knowledge in order to maintain his wholeness. The concepts of independence and need satisfaction have yet to be the object of the rigorous scientific scrutiny that is necessary to produce the knowledge required for nursing. What, indeed, is known about the elderly person's need to play? What descriptive studies have furnished information about the pregnant teenager's need to communicate? What research has experimented with strategies to supplement the motivation of cancer victims with regard to their need to learn to live with their illness?

Nurses who adopt another nursing frame of reference will also seek knowledge necessary for the practice of nursing. Not everyone has to have the same conceptual departure point. If knowledge developed by the "independence" school of thought should prove in conflict with that developed by the "behavioral equilibrium" (Johnson) or the "adaptation" (Roy) school of thought, more research would be stimulated and nursing science would push forward to new frontiers (Adam, 1987).

As nursing science advances, the utility of conceptual models will be examined: utility for planning client care, utility for developing curricula and for identifying research problems. The conceptual model for nursing that inspired the research in the first place may ultimately be judged less socially congruent, significant, and useful than had been expected. All will not be lost by any means; the knowledge gained will not be invalidated. But the conceptual base itself might have to be broadened, narrowed, or altered in some way. It might be replaced by another, which, in time, might also be found wanting.

Nurse scientists, as indeed all nurses, have some conception of nursing, acknowledged or not, specific to nursing or borrowed, explicit or implicit. Attempts to advance nursing science from a borrowed or unclear frame of reference surely involve more risks than would the same attempts from a conception complete enough to be called a conceptual model.

Phillips (1977) makes a strong case for conceptual models in the advancement of nursing science. Henderson's way of looking at nursing is one such conceptual model, and the prospect of constructing nursing science on the scaffolding of independence nursing seems as exciting as it is challenging.

person, environment, health, nursing

Discussions of nursing theory and nursing science bring to mind the importance given, in some instances, to four concepts and the links between them.

The concepts of person, environment, health, and nursing have been called the paradigm of nursing (Flaskerud & Halloran, 1980) and the metaparadigm of nursing (Fawcett, 1989). Jennings & Meleis (1988) accept the four concepts as the major features of the nursing paradigm but suggest five domain concepts: person, environment, health, interaction, and transition. Yeo (1989) refers to human beings, nurse, health, and environment (society) as the "key definitions of nursing theory" (p. 36), and Kim (1983) names client, environment, and nursing action as the domains of nursing.

Other authors (Downs, 1988; Ellis, see Pressler & Fitzpatrick, 1988; Leininger, see Rosenbaum, 1986; Peplau, 1988) seriously question the importance given to person, environment, health, and nursing as the elements of the discipline's focus.

Conceptions of nursing that have the structure of a conceptual model (assumptions, values, and major units) have been analyzed using the structure of person, environment, health, and nursing, and have been found wanting in their development of health and environment (Fawcett, 1989; Fitzpatrick & Whall, 1989).

The intent of a conceptual model is to conceptualize nursing as a discipline—nursing's specific contribution *to* health, nursing's particular responsibility *for* the environment. To consider person-as-client as part of a conception of nursing is obvious; to place "nursing" in a conception of nursing seems peculiarly redundant. But seeking development of the concepts "health" and "environment" in a conception of nursing may be searching for content that was not meant to be included. Health and environment are certainly of very great importance to nursing and to all health disciplines. Indeed, if the word "nursing" were replaced with "medicine" or "physiotherapy" or another health profession, the four concepts could easily constitute the meta-paradigm of that discipline.

This writer does not question the statement that the concepts of person, environment, health, and nursing make up nursing's metaparadigm. The same four concepts cannot, however, be the elements of nursing's paradigm (conceptual model for nursing).

Nurses committed to independence nursing must have considerable knowledge of health and of the environment; both are extremely complex and warrant much study and reflection. As for their conception of their own service to society, those nurses see the *person*-as-client as a complex whole presenting fourteen fundamental needs from which spring specific needs. They consider their particular contribution to *health* as the maintaining and restoring of client independence in need satisfaction. Their responsibility for the *environment* is present at every step of the systematic process: collection of data includes data about the environment; identification of many specific needs is directly related to physical and emotional environment; the complementing and supplementing of client strength is very often done by reducing environmental influences. For independence nurses, *nursing* as a discipline is conceptualized with the assumptions, values and major units of the Henderson model; *nursing* as intervention is the complementing-supplementing of client strength, will, or knowledge, with the short-term objective of need satisfaction and the middle- or long-term purpose of helping the client recover his independence in need satisfaction, or helping him toward a peaceful death.

Nursing education has long accorded great importance to "person"; courses in biology, physiology, pathology, psychology, sociology, anthropology, and others attest to that importance. Various courses in ecology and health are also given space in the curriculum. As for *nursing* courses, they are directly related to and dependent on the conception of nursing on which the programme is based.

To practise independence nursing, one must have knowledge of many concepts: health, environment, pain, grief and mourning, death, group dynamics and many others. Inasmuch as the phenomenon named in the concept is likely to influence client independence in need satisfaction, it is incumbent on the nurse to learn about it and thus improve her professional service to society.

chapter 14

adopting a conceptual model:
a planned change

The change that necessarily occurs when one adopts a conceptual model specific to nursing is the subject of this chapter. For some, it is indeed a radical change to embrace a conceptual model with its various implications for nursing education, practice and research, while for others it is, if anything, a simple change of vocabulary, since the model does not represent a substantial change.

This book is based on the premise that our private or personal way of conceptualizing nursing is not often clear and precise enough to be easily communicated to others. Our mental image of our profession is often so blurred that it cannot be understood, and such a lack of conceptual clarity is reflected in our way of being a nurse.

The change in question, first individual and then collective, consists in making our mental representation of nursing clear and explicit, in making precise what is now vague and ambiguous. To the extent that our present conception of nursing is difficult to express in words, the adoption of a complete and explicit conception represents an important change.

In the preceding chapters, one such complete and explicit way of looking at nursing has been described. It may correspond, in general, to the conception that many members of the profession already have; they might have perhaps liked to use the same words to define their goals and role but their idea was not quite as clear-cut as that of Virginia Henderson. Other nurses will react in a similar way to other conceptual models, remarking that the model indicates exactly what they have always believed or felt about nursing, but that words failed them to say so in such a clear and distinct manner. In all such instances, the model is merely the verbal expression of a concept already formed or in the process of being developed in the nurse's mind.

The change to be brought about is therefore minor or important, according to each nurse, but adopting a specific conceptual model is always a planned and deliberate change. A planned change is in opposition to one that occurs spontaneously, such as a change in the weather, or an inner change in personal attitudes or feelings that is not consciously planned.

To change, according to the dictionaries, is to alter by substituting something else for, to make different; change is the substitution of one thing in the place of another, any alteration.

A planned personal change of the inner self is frequently a long and painful process. It can be frightening to examine one's interior motives and to question one's mode of being, and while the end result may be positive, the actual process of changing is not always happy and carefree.

The same is true of a planned professional change, individual or collective. The prospect of giving up a certain way of being a nurse and substituting a more precise way is also a frightening and almost dangerous proposal, since there is no guarantee that the end result will be to everyone's entire satisfaction. Not all nurses are willing to take the risk; some are even convinced that there is no risk involved in *avoiding* change.

Change is, of course, a part of life, and it seems that all things are constantly changing. Heraclitus' philosophy suggests that everything is in a state of flux. Yet many things seem stable, even immovable. Lewin (1961) describes the conditions for "no change" as a state of quasi-stationary equilibrium. Those who resist the idea of change attempt to maintain the state of equilibrium, even though the stability is illusory; those who wish to implement change decry the same equilibrium. Both parties are heard to say that the more things change, the more they remain the same!

Let us imagine that a group of nurses, for example, in a school of nursing, health centre or hospital, are quite convinced that they must adopt a specific conceptual model in order to make clear the nature of their particular service to society. How should they go about implementing the change? How can they substitute one way of being a nurse for another and more precise way?

A planned change warrants long and earnest consideration. The various theories of change are beyond the scope of this book; the reader may consult the many texts devoted to the subject. Change experts describe diverse ways of conceptualizing change, the different strategies at the change-agent's disposal and the various kinds of resistance to change that are most often encountered (Bennis, Benne & Chin, 1969).

Most authors point out that for a change to be lasting, it must be brought about slowly. In the adoption of a conceptual model for nursing, it may be useful to discriminate five steps which, while not entirely separate one from the other, follow each other chronologically. The five steps are:

1. the sensitization period
2. the choice of the model
3. the study of the model
4. the adoption of the model
5. the stabilization period

In spite of the overlapping, each step is worth studying separately. The time required to accomplish each step may vary from a few weeks to several years.

the sensitization period

The first step in the long process of bringing about a lasting change is *to create the desire for change* by making all concerned individuals at all levels of the organization undergoing the change process aware of their wish to change or by actively intervening to create a wish to change. In other words, the change-agent, who may be one person or a group of persons, tries to portray the conceptual model as more desirable and more advantageous than the status quo which is depicted as being undesirable and disadvantageous. As long as the nurses are satisfied with the existing situation, they are hardly interested in changing. An important preliminary step is therefore that of increasing their awareness of their dissatisfaction, or that of creating discontent by extolling the merits of the conceptual model. "The place to begin change is at those points in the system where some stress and strain exist." (Benne & Birnbaum, 1969, p. 332)

The change-agent begins therefore, at the risk of being accused of subversive activities and of creating dissension in the group, to disturb the established order of things—that apparent stability that is maintained because the forces favourable to a specific model are equal to the opposing forces. Referring to Lewin's state of "no change," the driving forces are equal to the restraining forces; the quasi-equilibrium of the force field is maintained because the forces against change are equal to those that are for change. (Jenkins, 1961) The change-agent attempts to disturb the balance between the opposing forces. To do so he must identify each one of the forces. For this discussion, the driving forces favourable to the adoption of a conceptual model might be patients' complaints about their nursing care or the students' grievances concerning the curriculum, and the restraining forces could be distrust toward the change-agent or lack of time for discussion meetings owing to a heavy work load.

During the period of sensitization, each new argument proposed in favour of adopting a conceptual model results in a resisting counter-argument. The change-agent must recognize the importance of exploring carefully the nature of the resistance, listening attentively to all resisters and encouraging all expressions of hostility toward the model.

It should be recognized that resistance to change is something positive. It obliges the change-agent to double his efforts and strengthen his arguments, and resistance also keeps a change-committee from moving too quickly or omitting any phase of the process. Resistance may persuade the committee that the time is not ripe for the adoption of a conceptual model; in certain circumstances a delay can be beneficial to all concerned. The resisters may even succeed in convincing the change-committee that the status quo is to be preferred. In such a case, the change committee will abandon their project since it is obviously not the opportune moment, in that setting, to pursue the adoption of a conceptual model specific to nursing.

The opposition of the resisters engenders a number of interesting questions: Why are nurses reluctant to have their social mission clearly defined? Where is the danger in making explicit the nature of nursing's service to society? Would an unequivocal professional identity perhaps oblige us to assume our responsibilities and act, collectively, as adults rather than adolescents? Is it possible that determining, even in abstract terms, the scope of our role in society would hold us accountable for a specific service rather than for "nothing special, most anything and a little of everything"?*

Complaints coming from patients, students, and the general public are often discussed at length, without anyone questioning the purpose and identity of nursing. In the same way, grievances expressed by administrative or governmental authorities are often explained away without referring to the lack of clarity in the role of the nurse. Without simplifying every problem by calling it an identity crisis, the change-agent can bring such fundamental questions into any discussion of problems about nursing practice or education.

The legitimate fear of too much precision may be a form of resistance to a conceptual model. Nurses insist, and rightly so, on protecting their autonomy and they resist any attempt to force them to follow a recipe. But the conceptual model is an abstraction; it cannot be a recipe book. The link between the abstract and the concrete is furnished by the nurse who, bringing to bear her own creativeness, intuition, and individuality, uses the systematic process (based on her conceptual model) to discover concrete interventions to help the client. A precise

---

* The writer is indebted to a former student for this résumé of the role of nursing.

mental image of nursing can even stimulate creative activity since a unifying goal encourages the professional commitment of the group members.

Other nurses may resist the idea of accepting someone's "definition of nursing"; further explanation may convince them that a conceptual model *for* nursing is a conception of what nursing could or should be. A definition will be possible the day when nurses can say that nursing is that which, today, they can merely say it could or should be. Some others may resist the idea of "teaching untested theory"; the change-agent will have to return to distinctions between theories and conceptual models.

When the majority of people concerned see the change, with all the risks it entails, as preferable to the present state of "no change," the time has come to begin the actual change. When nurse administrators, educators, practitioners and researchers realize that they are not too sure of what they should teach and research, question what nursing care really is, and find out that they are disconcerted by that confusion, the period of sensitization is drawing to a close. The change-committee can now turn to the choice of the conceptual model.

the choice of the model

The great majority of nurses in the group are now sincerely committed to adopting a conceptual model. But which model? A decision of such importance is not to be taken lightly; it may be made by several methods.

1. A committee, or a small group, may choose for the others. Among the existing models, they will choose the simplest or the most complex, the most familiar or the least known, according to group preference. Other considerations are the model's usefulness for education, practice and research, the expectations of society with regard to the nursing profession and the significance for the clients of the kind of nursing care that follows from the model. The committee's decision is submitted to a larger group for approval.

2. Each individual person participates in the choice. The committee plans ways and means by which everyone can engage in a comparative study of several models so that an informed choice can be made.

Both of the above two ways of making the choice are lengthy processes; however, the second has the advantage of assuring everyone's participation in the decision. In the end, the change will be more lasting if every concerned person has been part of the decision-making process. Accepting a decision imposed by others often means a short-lived allegiance!

3. The committee, or the entire group, develops its own conceptual model for nursing. The great advantage of such an undertaking is the personal investment of each participant which increases the subsequent acceptance of the change. However, Stevens (1979) warns against the difficulties of group endeavours when the task is one of conceptualizing. The author of a conceptual model makes use of her insight and intuition as well as a rational and scientific approach; conceptualizing as a group may make the use of individual insight and experience very difficult. Choosing a theory from which to draw the assumptions would not be an easy group decision; making explicit the value system and identifying the six major units are tasks for which group consensus would not come easily.

While the new model is being developed, schools of nursing do not usually close down, nor do hospitals and other care agencies cease to function. Yet the care that is still being given and the nursing that is still being taught must necessarily be based on *something*. Can people committed to clarity and precision continue to teach or practise in the absence of a solid conceptual base? Obviously, a compromise must be found.

4. The group chooses one of the existing conceptual models for the immediate future and plans to begin the development of the new and original model.

A fifth possibility that seems to interest at least some nurses is to take a part of each of the existing models and from the parts forge a new "eclectic" model. This writer cannot recommend such a procedure; the existing models are based on assumptions that differ greatly from model to model, and to choose bits and pieces from several models would only jeopardize the theoretical foundation of the "new" model. Its internal logic and consistency would be endangered and its clarity and precision threatened. It will be recalled that practice, education and research are to be based on a conception of nursing that is clear and precise.

the study of the model

Once the model has been chosen, either by all interested individuals, or by a committee with subsequent approval by the majority, an exhaustive study of the model must be undertaken. It is already somewhat known, since it has been chosen from among others, but a study in more depth is now necessary in order to master all its subtleties. Readings, lectures, workshops, discussions, consultations, and so forth are useful in helping all interested parties understand the assumptions, values, major units, and implications of the model.

At this stage new forms of resistance can emerge. It is entirely positive that dissenters openly express their objections at this step in the process, as at all others. Unspoken reservations may later bring about the sabotage of the model by the people who give it lip service only.

This third step is long and may be difficult, but the time and energy spent at this point may save time later on. If the nurses at all levels of the organization have not integrated the concepts and sub-concepts of the model or adopted the terminology of the model (*i.e.*, if they have not made their mental image of nursing the same as that of the model), it would become difficult, if not impossible, to go on to the next step, the adoption stage.

the adoption

A way of looking at, or conceptualizing, nursing can only be adopted in one place: the mind's eye of the nurse. The change-agent can, of course, do much to facilitate that implantation or inculcation in the minds of others: providing the working instruments (assessment tool, care plan), using the vocabulary of the model, valuing the concepts of the model, rewarding any evidence that the systematic process is indeed based on the model, etc.

It is often forgotten that the conception of nursing on which many educators, practitioners, and researchers currently base their teaching, nursing care and research (for those activities are always based on *some* mental image) was never "implanted" or "adopted" in systematic fashion. No one ever announced that, beginning on a certain date, nurses would have to adopt that conception. Yet that way of conceptualizing nursing is very solidly in place in the minds of nurses; in fact, it is so deeply rooted that nurses resist the idea of replacing it with one distinct to nursing. If the current conception is so taken for granted, it may be because its vocabulary has long been used, its concepts have long been valued and actions based on it have long been those that were rewarded. If indeed that conception was ever "imposed" on nurses, it was done in very subtle fashion.

Today's change agents may find it wise to proceed in an equally unobtrusive way. If words and actions consistent with the conceptual model could gradually and discreetly become the words and actions that are valued and rewarded, the change will take place in the minds and in the behaviour of those concerned.

Whatever the setting where change is desired, the conceptual model is not *added to* the existing conceptual base. The planned change consists in exchanging the current frame of reference for one that warrants the name "conceptual model for nursing". The current way of looking at nursing is often a medical one; acknowledged or not, the medical model, an eminently useful one for physicians, is often the nurse's frame of reference also. Adopting a conceptual framework specific to nursing means replacing the "medical vision of nursing" with a "nursing vision of nursing".

the stabilization period

When the conceptual base is established and all activities are animated by it, the process of planned change has not ended; a period of watchfulness is necessary to insure that the new guidelines are solidly in place (Lewin's refreezing). Follow-up discussions and problem-solving sessions are useful to keep people from slipping back to the former way of looking at nursing. More or less consciously, we tend to return to the former and less demanding conceptual framework.

The stabilization period may also be used to inform schools, hospitals and any others who might be interested, about the change. Members of the health team that work most closely with the nurses involved in the change should be included in some of the discussion, so that all who work for the good of the client will understand that the nurses have a precise way of conceptualizing their contribution to the client's health. Incredulous outcries or disdainful remarks may require patient and tactful clarification, but there is nothing like self-confidence (personal or professional) to help one assert oneself constructively; a sure identity and the strength of one's convictions help considerably when one wishes to take one's rightful place in the world.

Perhaps a word of caution against unrealistic expectations should be entered here. The adoption of a conceptual model will not solve all of nursing's problems. It cannot provide more than it is meant to provide: a clear and explicit way of conceptualizing our service to society. The model does not tell us what to do nor how to perform techniques and procedures; it only indicates, in abstract terms, the type of intervention, without spelling out the intervention itself. If the model dictated the actions of the nurse, it would not *be* a conceptual model, but rather a book of recipes. Nor will the adoption of a specific frame of reference turn poor communication skills and ineffective interpersonal relationships into empathic interactions. Where a helping relationship already exists, a conceptual model can only improve it.

In the long run, the group of nurses initiating the change process may realize they have not chosen well nor wisely. At the long-term evaluation, that is, after several years, the model may prove to be less socially useful, significant and congruent than was hoped. The group will then choose another model—perhaps one that has demonstrated its advantages elsewhere. The experience with the first one is far from lost, for the group will have learned to be more demanding and discriminating and will shrewdly seek even more clarity and precision in their new model.

Adopting a conceptual model does not have to be a life-long commitment. It is serious commitment which deserves our support and confidence, but after several years of honest effort we do not have to remain bound to one model if another one seems more useful.

To adopt a conceptual model, specific to our profession, simply affords us a precise way of looking at nursing and therefore clear direction for those who choose, or have chosen, to be a nurse.

chapter 15

clinical examples

Three fictitious situations illustrate independence nursing.

example a

Mrs. Mary Brown, aged 58, is admitted by stretcher to her hospital room. She comes directly from the emergency room where she was examined by the physician. Her chart is still in emergency. During the transfer from stretcher to bed, the nurse makes a brief assessment, relying on direct observation, since Mrs. Brown seems unable to answer questions. The collection of data, necessarily incomplete, yields the following information:

Eat and drink: _____

Breathe: respiration quiet, 18/min

Eliminate:
— incontinent of urine
— profuse diaphoresis

Move and maintain desirable postures:
— does not move R side, R side flaccid
— moves L side often, nervously
— L side of mouth pulled downward

Sleep and rest: drowsy at times

Dress and undress: _____

Maintain T°: 37°C

Keep clean: hair, skin, nails in excellent condition

Avoid dangers:
— fall from bed
— contractures of R side
— skin irritation (incontinence)
— extreme anxiety

Communicate:	— very alert at times
	— speaks unintelligibly
	— eyes anxious
	— gestures nervously with L hand
Worship:	— rosary held in L hand
	— religious medal attached to wrist-watch
Work ...:	_____
Play ...:	_____
Learn ...:	_____

The nurse plans to complete the assessment when the family arrives; she will consult the medical file and the physician's orders as soon as they arrive. But even with data collection incomplete, she begins the second step of the systematic process: the identification of Mrs. Brown's specific needs.

1. voids, in bedpan, 6-7 times daily
2. moves R arm and leg at least 4 times daily
3. changes position q. 2 h
4. keeps R arm and leg in functional position
5. washes herself in bed
6. — avoids contractures of R side
   — avoids falling out of bed
   — avoids skin breakdown
   — avoids staying alone for long periods (anxiety)
7. communicates anxiety, needs
8. — keeps rosary at hand
   — receives visit from priest

Continuing the second step of the systematic process, the nurse decides if the specific needs are satisfied and if not, why not. Then, in the third step, she plans the focus and mode of intervention as well as the complementary-supplementary action.

For each of the specific needs, the nurse reasons as follows:

need #1

— not satisfied because of lack of strength (cortical control of sphinctre, control of speech)
— intervention focus: sphinctre control, speech control
— intervention mode: substitute
— action: — offer bedpan q. 2-3 h
    — be attentive to non-verbal indications of desire to void

need #2

— not satisfied because of lack of strength
— intervention focus: muscular strength of R side
— intervention mode: replace
— action: — passive range-of-motion exercises 9-13-18 h.s.
    — as soon as feasible, show her how to use her L hand for passive exercises to R arm

need #3

— not satisfied owing to lack of strength of R side
— intervention focus: — muscular strength R side
        — muscular strength L side
— intervention mode: — substitute for strength of R side
        — reinforce strength of L side
— action: — turn her from side to side q. 2 h
    — encourage her to use L side and bedrails to help turn herself

need #4

— not satisfied, related to lack of strength
— intervention focus: muscular strength of R side
— intervention mode: reinforce strength
— action: place R hand, arm, leg in functional position (cushions, rolls, etc.) at each change of position

need #5

— not satisfied, related to lack of strength of R arm

— intervention focus: muscular strength of R arm
— intervention mode: substitute for strength
— action: — place toilet articles within reach of L hand
　　　　　 — complete bath (L side, back, legs, etc.)
　　　　　 — lanolin massage (pressure points, incontinence)

need #6

— not satisfied because of lack of strength
— intervention focus: muscular strength of R side
— intervention mode: substitute for strength
— action: — see needs #2, 3, 4, 5
　　　　　 — bedrails up
　　　　　 — see need #7

need #7

— not satisfied, related to lack of strength (cortical control) and
　insufficient knowledge (how to compensate)
— intervention focus: — speech control
　　　　　　　　　　 — knowledge of non-verbal communica-
　　　　　　　　　　　 tion
— intervention mode: — substitute for cortical control
　　　　　　　　　　 — add to knowledge of non-verbal means
— action: — validate (verbally) the meaning of her gestures
　　　　　 — speak slowly; check her understanding
　　　　　 — call-bell within reach of L hand. Explain its use
　　　　　 — be attentive to her facial expressions
　　　　　 — acknowledge her anxiety
　　　　　 — return to her frequently
　　　　　 — explain all care measures

need #8

— not satisfied because of lack of strength
— intervention focus: strength of R side
— intervention mode: substitute for strength
— action: — place rosary within reach of L hand
　　　　　 — notify priest (daily list)

The immediate care plan for Mrs. Brown begins as follows:

specific need	nurse's action
(client necessity)	(complementing-supplementing)
1. voids, in bedpan, 6-7 times daily	— offer bedpan q. 2-3 h — be attentive to non-verbal indications of desire to void
2. moves R arm and leg at least 4 times daily	— passive range-of-motion exercises 9-13-18-h.s. — as soon as feasible, show her how to use L hand for passive exercises to R arm

When the physician's orders arrive, need #1 is changed to: through indwelling catheter, passes at least 400 cc of clear yellow urine q. 8 h. This specific need (a necessity for Mrs. Brown) is somewhat passive, but it is certainly a necessary activity for Mrs. Brown. The need must therefore be satisfied. Mrs. Brown cannot, is not able to, satisfy the need on her own; it is therefore a case of insufficient strength—strength to take in enough fluids, to care for the catheter, etc. (No doubt Mrs. Brown lacks knowledge about catheter care, but it is hardly reasonable to expect her to know such techniques. She may have to learn them later; for the moment, it is not due to her lack of knowledge if at least 400 cc of urine do not pass through her catheter every eight hours.) As well as substituting for Mrs. Brown's strength (forcing fluids, aseptic care of the catheter, unclamping the catheter, etc.), the nurse will recognize new "dangers" to be avoided: loss of bladder-muscle tone and urinary infection.

The physician's orders include "liquids only: 2000-3000 cc daily". Mrs. Brown's specific need will be: drinks at least 1200 cc (day), 600 cc (evening) and 200 cc (night). Mrs. Brown does not satisfy this need on her own; it must therefore be satisfied with the complementing-supplementing actions of the nurse. If Mrs. Brown does not have enough will (impaired vitality) to drink 2000-3000 cc of liquid, the nurse will seek to increase her motivation to do so. As well, Mrs. Brown lacks strength (left facial muscles, right hand and arm). To substitute for that strength, the nurse may hold the drinking straw in the right side of Mrs. Brown's mouth while she holds the glass for her, offering her small quantities at a time of her preferred juice.

In carrying out her interventions, the fourth step of the process, the nurse uses Maslow's hierarchy of needs to help her establish priority among the many personal needs identified for Mrs. Brown. The patient's vital functions are not in danger and some personal needs are still not identified. The nurse intervenes to help satisfy Mrs. Brown's more physiological needs, all the while paying special attention to her need to communicate. All efforts to satisfy any of the patient's needs will include interventions to satisfy need #7. At each contact with Mrs. Brown the nurse will try to establish and maintain a helping relationship by communicating her empathy, authenticity, and so forth.

The fifth step of the process, the evaluation, is left to the reader's imagination. Interventions that prove to be ineffective in satisfying the identified needs will be replaced by others, and interventions that prove helpful will be maintained. The entire process is repeated, as necessary, with a view to restoring, or in some instances at least maintaining, Mrs. Brown's independence in satisfying all her needs.

It will be noted that the care planned for Mrs. Brown is not highly individual; the personal needs that have been identified could be those of many other people in a similar situation, although they are far from being the needs of every human being. The assessment is still incomplete. As Mrs. Brown and her family provide more information, the care plan will be more individualized. Meanwhile, the fact that Mrs. Brown's specific or individual needs are not *unique* does not release the nurse from the obligation to note them on the care plan so that all nursing personnel (day, evening and night staff) maintain the care during the twenty-four hour period.

Some days later, Mrs. Brown's neurological condition worsens and the medical staff perform a tracheotomy. With regard to the fundamental need to breathe, Mrs. Brown's specific or particular need is now as follows:

— with the help of a tracheostomy, breathes quietly 18-24 times/min; breathes humidified air.

The lack of respiratory strength (for humidifying air, coughing, expectorating) calls for various complementing-supplementing actions by the nurse. They were all learned as "technique for tracheotomy care"; she now sees them as a means of satisfying Mrs. Brown's specific need.

This recent change in Mrs. Brown's condition calls for the identification of other specific needs related to communicating, learning, and drinking.

Before leaving Mrs. Brown's nursing care plan it will be noted that the client's needs have been entered on the care plan using verbs in the present tense; the form is easy and indicates that the needs are very much of *the present time*. However, the nurses' preference may be to put all verbs in the future tense or in the infinitive form. She may prefer to write them as objectives and she may even write "nurse's objectives" in a column between the client objectives and the nurse's actions. The precise formula to be used may vary from one setting to another. What is paramount, whatever the setting, is that Mrs. Brown's needs are clearly indicated as well as the nursing interventions that will help satisfy them, all with the intent of restoring the client's independence in satisfying her own needs.

example b

Harold Green, 22, is an outpatient. His diagnosis: depressive reaction. A student nurse, beginning her clinical experience in that setting, chooses to follow Harold.

After her first encounter with him at the clinic, she summarizes the data she collected.

Eat and drink:	— poor appetite
	— eats very quickly without tasting anything
	— does not notice what he eats
	— has no likes and dislikes
	— knows he is too thin (1.6 m, 50 kg)
	— no wine, no alcohol
Breathe:	— smokes two packages a day and would like to stop smoking
Eliminate:	— 7-8 micturitions a day
	— bowels move once a day; if constipated, takes a laxative—needs one, two or three times a week
	— considers regularity important
Move ...:	— no sports, no physical exercise
	— comes to the clinic by bus
	— holds himself straight, hands clenched, face tense
Sleep and rest:	— sleeps about 4 h/night in spite of medication (prescribed by physician)
	— when awake, feels tense and anxious
	— has occasional bad dreams
	— wakens early each morning but often stays in bed until 9 or 10 o'clock
	— is convinced nothing can be done
Dress and undress:	is not interested in clothes; wears clean jeans, gold chain
Maintain T°:	says he usually feels chilly; dresses accordingly
Keep clean:	— has a shower daily by force of habit
	— not interested in grooming
	— hair, nails are clean
Avoid dangers:	— afraid he will end up abandoning the clinic
	— afraid he will not keep appointments with his therapist

	— does not see any way a nurse can help
Communicate:	— reports a "good" relationship with his sister and brother-in-law, with whom he lives
	— says he talks to them little; has difficulty talking to people. Would like to be able to talk to his sister
	— explains he has never been able to talk to people. Has no friends. Has had no girlfriend for two years
	— calls himself a "loner"
	— seems wary of the nurse
	— wonders why the therapist bothers with him
Worship:	— has not practised for several years (educated as Roman Catholic)
	— reads oriental philosophy
Work:	— dropped out of university two years ago
	— does not work
	— declares himself lacking in ambition. (In his chart, a long and detailed social history describes Harold's perception of his life: an irreversible failure)
Play:	— reads a great deal
	— no longer goes to movies or ball games
	— feels he never really relaxes
	— sometimes plays with his sister's baby of 18 months
Learn:	— in reply to a question "what would you like to learn about your health?", he asks "what is the meaning of life?"
	— declares himself in "excellent health. I'm just depressed"

The student identifies Harold's individual needs with his help and participation. Several of his specific needs, in the areas of cleanliness, temperature, clothing, and religion for example, while identified during this second step of the systematic process, are not mentioned on the care plan. Harold is independent in the satisfaction of such needs and the nurse's intervention is not required, not even to maintain his independence. The needs that are noted on the care plan are as follows:

1. improve appetite, eat more slowly
2. reduce smoking by 1 cigarette a day
3. reduce use of laxatives
4. walk thirty minutes daily
5. sleep at least 6-7 h/night
6. express his feelings about himself, about his treatment
7. make friends (male and female)
8. learn to talk to his sister

The student plans to discuss with the physician the number of sleeping pills Harold is taking. She will discuss with the entire therapeutic team her nursing care plan.

For each specific need identified, the student continues the systematic process with Harold's participation.

need #1

— not satisfied independently, related to insufficient motivation and knowledge
— intervention focus: — motivation to eat slowly
                       — knowledge of how to increase appetite
— intervention mode: — increase motivation and knowledge
— action: — explore with him his habit of hurrying at the table
           — discuss the meaning of food for him
           — suggest he try to talk during the meal
           — suggest he ask his sister to prepare something he likes
           — explain the effects of exercise as appetizer, of play as appetizer (relaxation)

need #2

— not satisfied independently, related to insufficient will and knowledge

— intervention focus: — motivation to cut down smoking
                        — knowledge of methods
— intervention mode: — reinforce motivation
                        — complete knowledge
— action: — discuss with him his reasons for wanting to stop
            — plan with him which smoking periods will be
              eliminated each day
            — suggest new strategies (substitutes, "I quit" group,
              etc.)

need #3

— not satisfied independently owing to insufficient knowledge
— intervention focus: knowledge of ways to avoid laxatives
— intervention mode: add to his knowledge
— action: — explain effects of exercise on peristalsis
            — explain importance of liquids, fibre foods

need #4

— not satisfied independently owing to lack of motivation
— intervention focus: will to exercise more
— intervention mode: increase his motivation
— action: — explore with him his tendency to inactivity, what
              it obtains for him
            — verify if part of the trip to the clinic could be
              made on foot
            — remind him of relationship between exercise and
              appetite, sleeping, elimination

need #5

— not satisfied independently owing to lack of strength to combat
  tension and lack of knowledge of how to change his sleeping
  habits
— intervention focus: — strength to overcome tension
                        — knowledge of good sleeping habits
— intervention mode: — increase strength by reducing tension
                        — increase knowledge

— action: — explore with him ways of relaxing before bedtime (physical exercise, *light* reading, breathing exercises, etc.)
            — explain relationship between exercise, diet and sleeping patterns
            — encourage him to get up at a regular hour

need #6

— not satisfied independently, related to lack of motivation
— intervention focus: motivation to express his feelings
— intervention mode: increase his motivation
— action: — listen carefully, demonstrate warmth, respect, understanding
            — avoid interpretations, judgements
            — avoid getting into "philosophical" discussions, keep attention on his feelings
            — find out what he expects of the nurse
            — begin and end each encounter on time

need #7

— not satisfied independently, related to lack of motivation
— intervention focus: motivation to make friends
— intervention mode: increase his motivation
— action: — explore what his "loner" habits obtain for him
            — discuss with him how he would go about it, if he decided to make friends

need #8

— not satisfied independently, owing to insufficient motivation
— intervention focus: motivation to talk to his sister
— intervention mode: reinforce his motivation
— action: begin by exploring with him what he would like to say to his sister

Harold is in complete agreement that the identified needs are his requirements. The non-satisfaction of many of them is related to insufficient will. He wants to, but he doesn't dare; he wants to but not enough; he wants to but does not want to at the same time. When strength is lacking, Harold can't satisfy his need and when he has insufficient knowledge, he does not know how. At each encounter with Harold, the student adds to her collection of data and modifies specific needs and interventions accordingly.

example c

Mrs. Jean White, aged 27, is visited in her home by a community health nurse. The client has two children: Nancy, 2½ years, and Tommy, 5 months. For the third time since Tommy's birth, Mrs. White has had an episode of acute cystitis, treated successfully the preceding times with penicillin. The nurse summarizes the data from the initial interview:

Eat and drink:	— is delighted to have returned to her normal weight
	— eats well; feels it is very important to do so
	— well-informed about the vitamin and mineral content, etc. of food
	— drinks 10-12 glasses of liquid daily since taking penicillin
Breathe:	— does not smoke
	— concerned about environmental pollution
Eliminate:	— urinates 8-10 times a day, 2-3 times each night
	— burning sensation on micturition has lessened since penicillin treatment begun
	— bowel movements regular, daily
Move ...:	active in sports (skiing, swimming, walking)
Sleep and rest:	— sleeps well, except for getting up to void
	— manages to rest during the day
Dress and undress:	well dressed, fashion conscious

Maintain T°:   checks T° daily since beginning of infection (remains 37°C)

Keep clean:
— prefers a tub bath each evening but has a shower because of the infection
— after each voiding and bowel movement, is careful not to contaminate the urinary meatus
— breasts in good condition. Breast fed baby for 4 months
— children, house are clean

Avoid dangers:
— is anxious to avoid another infection, fears long-term complications
— wants to avoid a third pregnancy for 2-3 years
— fears she may be somehow responsible for the infections

Communicate:
— is very happy with her husband. They both want a third child; at present uses a diaphragm
— shares her concerns about the infection with her husband, who is very supportive
— admits her frustration about her infections, is pleased to talk to a nurse

Worship: with her husband, is an active member of the Anglican church

Work:
— feels her work as mother and homemaker is very important
— plans to return to her work as a physiotherapist at some later date
— active in church activities
— enjoys reading, TV, fresh air sports
— has many friends
— movies, theatre 2-3 times a month
— feels it is important to have evenings out with her husband

Learn: — wants to read, learn "everything" about prevention and treatment of bladder infections
                         — requests references about the psychogenesis of infections

With Mrs. White's enthusiastic participation, the nurse identifies several specific needs. Those that require no nursing action, neither to maintain nor restore independence, are left to Mrs. White's efficient management. Those entered on the care plan are:

1. to continue voiding 8-10 times a day
2. to avoid getting up at night to void
3. to continue expressing her fears about her repeated infections
4. to learn about infections (causes, treatments)

The nurse and Mrs. White continue. If the specific needs are not satisfied independently, why not? Is it that Mrs. White *can't* satisfy them, "won't" satisfy them, or does not know how? What should be the nurse's focus and mode of intervention? What action should she take?

need #1

— satisfied independently. There is no dependency problem. The nurse's intervention is to prevent a problem (maintain independence)
— intervention focus: maintaining independence
— intervention mode: reinforce will and knowledge
— action: — commend her efforts to force fluids
             — repeat importance of fluids (toxins, antibiotics)

need #2

— not satisfied. She can't. Lack of strength (bladder capacity vs inflammation and increased stimulation)
— intervention focus: bladder tolerance

— intervention mode: increase bladder tolerance by reducing stimulation
— action: suggest that her 12 glasses of liquid be re-distributed so as to drink less in the hours before bedtime

need #3

— satisfied independently. Independence must be maintained
— intervention focus: maintaining independence
— intervention mode: reinforce her motivation
— action: — listen attentively, avoid interpretations
            — encourage any expression of how she sees herself responsible
            — explore what an infection means to her
            — commend her willingness to talk openly

need #4

— not satisfied, related to lack of knowledge of where to obtain documentation
— intervention focus: knowledge of references
— intervention mode: add to knowledge
— action: — suggest available articles, books
            — ask what her physician has already told her
            — encourage her to ask him how to avoid another infection

The three preceding examples illustrate the systematic process based on Henderson's way of looking at nursing. Mrs. Brown had many dependency problems, while Harold and Mrs. White satisfied many of their specific needs independently. Whether the client is well or seriously ill, the nurse's social role is a complementary-supplementary one; she adds to his strength, will or knowledge in order to maintain, restore and promote his independence in need satisfaction.

In the three examples, a helping relationship is essential at every step of the systematic process. Technical skills, whether verbal or manual, are also necessary for effective intervention.

From the first to the last encounter with a given patient, knowledge of the human and biological sciences is imperative.

The carrying out of physicians' orders remains important; it is that part of nursing that is delegated. For the autonomous part of nursing, for the "more than that" (discussed in the Introduction to this book), a clear and explicit conception of nursing is mandatory.

Experienced nurses, of course, are able to plan and carry out effective interventions and, having intervened effectively, they can then justify their actions with scientific principles. Young nurses, whether students or new graduates, are, on the other hand, much less rich in experience, and they are hardly willing to wait until they have accumulated long years of experience before being able to provide effective nursing care. The three preceding examples demonstrate a process whereby the nurse who has clearly conceptualized her professional role has a substantive content and a rationale that will help her arrive at an appropriate intervention. The experience she gains with the years will be all the richer because it has been based on a conceptual model and her practice will contribute to the development of nursing science.

For nurses of any age group, a complete and explicit conception of their profession gives meaning to the entire systematic process, from the initial assessment to the evaluation. A precise way of looking at nursing constitutes a framework within which all professional activities, however disparate certain acts may seem, are oriented toward the goal that the nurse wishes to attain. Any beginning or experienced nurse who chooses to take advantage of such a framework may well discover not only a greater sense of professional commitment, but an increase in feelings of personal satisfaction.

appendix

assessment tool
for independence nursing

independence nursing assessment tool

Name of client: _____ Age: ___ Male: __ Female: __

Lives with: _____

Nationality (or ethnic group): _____

Medical Diagnosis: _____

Associated diagnoses: _____

Allergies: _____   Medications: _____

                                                     _____

                                                     _____

                                                     _____

                                                     _____

T.P.R.: _____   B.P.: _____

Eat and drink adequately

1. What is your daily eating routine? (number of meals, schedule, type of food)*

2. What do you drink in an ordinary day? (quantity, type ...)*

3. How has your ...** changed your routine?

4. Would you say you eat well or badly? Why do you say this?

---

* Words in brackets are intended to help the nurse ask additional questions if necessary. They are not meant to suggest answers.

** The nurse replaces ... with the most appropriate words: illness, health problem, accident or, more specifically, heart condition, bladder infection, arthritis, etc. If the client is well, the question is simply omitted.

5. How important is it to you that you (and your family) eat well? (very, somewhat, not important).

6. What are your particular likes and dislikes?

7. Under what conditions do you eat less well? (certain emotions, stress, overwork, weather).

8. What helps you most to eat well?

9. What special requirements do you have about eating and drinking? (help to prepare meals, special utensils).

    Nurse's observations (incl. weight, height):

Breathe normally

10. Ordinarily, would you describe your breathing as easy or difficult?

11. How has your ... affected your breathing?

12. What habits do you have that might affect your breathing? (smoking, position, environment, medication, yoga, etc.).

13. What importance do you attach to a clean environment?

14. Does your breathing change when you are anxious, worried or angry?

    Nurse's observations:

Eliminate body wastes

15. What are your voiding habits? (frequency, characteristics, stoma).

16. What seems to affect those habits? (medication, food, drink, emotions).

17. How has your ... changed your routine? (pain, position, etc.).

18. What have you found to be helpful?

19. How important is it to you to have regular voidings? (very, somewhat, not important).

20. What are your bowel habits? (frequency, type of stool, stoma).

21. What affects those habits? (food, drink, exercise, medication, emotions, cold).

22. How has your ... affected your routine? (pain, position, etc.).

23. How do you handle problems of constipation or diarrhea?

24. How important is it to you to have regular bowel habits? (very, somewhat, not important).

25. What special requirements do you have for bowel or bladder regularity? (solitude, calm, environmental props).

    Nurse's observations:

Move and maintain desirable postures

26. Would you describe yourself as physically active? Yes _____ No _____

27. What main activities do you have that require you to move about? (work, sports, exercise, travel).

28. How has your ... changed your habits?

29. What would prevent you from keeping up your activities? (pain, emotions, fatigue).

30. How do you handle pain, fatigue?

31. How important is it to you to keep up your physical activities? (very, somewhat, not important).

    Nurse's observations:

Sleep and rest

32. What is your usual sleep and rest routine? (number of hours, quality).

33. How has your ... changed this?

34. What sort of thing can disturb your sleep? (excitement, food, drink, loneliness, medication, pain).

35. What do you find helpful? (relaxation, music, time of retiring).

36. How important is it to you to have enough sleep and rest? (very, somewhat, not important).

    Nurse's observations:

Dress and undress

37. How has your ... affected your habits of dressing and undressing? (pain, limitations).

38. What special requirements do you have? (prosthesis, fashion).

39. How important is it to you to be "well-dressed", "in style"? (very, somewhat, not important).

    Nurse's observations:

Maintain body temperature

40. In general, how do you tolerate heat and cold, changes in temperature?

41. Has your ... changed this?

42. What special requirements do you have for keeping your temperature normal? (clothing, environment, emotional climate).

43. How do such emotions as happiness and excitement or anxiety and anger affect your temperature?

    Nurse's observations:

Keep the body clean and well groomed and protect the integument

44. What is your usual routine for keeping clean and caring for your skin, hair, nails, etc.? (shower, shampoo, dental care).

45. How has your ... changed this?

46. What special requirements do you have? (foot-care, prosthesis, stoma, genital hygiene),

47. How important is it to you to be clean and well-groomed? (very, somewhat, not important).

    Nurse's observations (incl. environment):

Avoid dangers and avoid injuring others

48. For your general safety, what situations or circumstances is it important for you to avoid? (allergy, medication, effort, infection).

49. For your peace of mind, what emotional situations are to be avoided? (certain persons, loneliness, fear).

50. How can a nurse help you avoid any of these dangers?

51. What special requirements do you have in order to avoid injuring or offending others? (prothesis, care of stoma, taking of medications, emotional climate).

    Nurse's observations:

Communicate with others in expressing emotions, needs, fears or opinions

52. Who is (are) the most important person(s) in your life? (child, parent, spouse, friend).

53. With what person(s) do you share problems and discuss ideas?

54. How does your ... change this?

55. In general, would you say you talk freely about your feelings or do you "hold things in"?

56. How important is it to you to share your concerns with someone? (very, somewhat, not important).

57. How do you feel about having to ask for help—from a nurse—from friends?

Nurse's observations:

Worship according to one's faith

58. In general, what requirements do you have because of your personal philosophy, your spiritual beliefs or your particular faith or religion? (food, meditation, attendance at service).

59. How has your ... changed this?

60. How important to you are your spiritual or religious beliefs? (very, somewhat, not important).

61. In regard to your health care, what might be questioned or forbidden because of those beliefs? (foods, medical treatment, abortion).

Nurse's observations:

Work in such a way that there is a sense of accomplishment

62. What is your main occupation? (work, school, home-making).

63. How important is that to you? (very, somewhat, not important).

64. How has your ... changed that?

65. What other activities that are important to you take up your time? (volunteer work, union activities, second job).

Nurse's observations:

Play or participate in various forms of recreation

66. What do you usually do to relax and enjoy yourself? (sports, reading, music).

67. How important is it to you to reserve some time for relaxing? (very, somewhat, not important).

68. How has your ... changed your methods of relaxing?

69. What benefits do you see in having some time "to play"?

Nurse's observations:

Learn, discover and use available health facilities

70. What would you like to learn about your health and about your family's health?

71. What do you know and what would you like to learn about your ...? your medications? your treatment?

72. How important is it to you to be well-informed about your own and your family's health? (very, somewhat, not important).

73. Where do you obtain information about health? (health professionals, media, books).

———————————————

— Is there anything you would like to talk to someone about?
— Of all the things we have just discussed, what seems most important to you at this time?
— I have no further questions for the moment. Do you have any questions, comments or remarks?

references

Abdellah, F.G. (1964). *Patient-centered approaches to nursing.* New York: Macmillan.

Adam, E. (1985). Toward more clarity in terminology: Frameworks, theories and models. *Journal of Nursing Education,* 24, 151-155.

Adam, E. (1987). Nursing theory: What it is and what it is not. *The Canadian Journal of Nursing Research (Nursing Papers),* 19 (1), 5-14.

Alderman, M.K. (1980). Self-responsibility in health-care promotion: Motivational factors. *Journal of School Health,* January, 22-25.

Anderson, J.E. & Briggs, L.L. (1988). Nursing diagnosis: A study of quality and supportive evidence. *Image: Journal of Nursing Scholarship,* 20 (3), 141-144.

Aspinall, M.J. (1976). Nursing diagnosis, the weak link. *Nursing Clinics of North America,* 10 (3), 449-460.

Becker, H.S. (1969). Personal change in adult life, In W.G. Bennis, R. Benne, R. Chin (Ed.), *The planning of change,* 2nd ed. (pp. 255-267). New York: Holt, Rinehart & Winston.

Benne, K.D. & Birnbaum, M. (1969). Principles of changing. In W.G. Bennis, R. Benne, R. Chin (Ed.), *The planning of change,* 2nd ed. (pp. 328-335). New York: Holt, Rinehart & Winston.

Bennis, W.G., Benne, R., Chin, R. (Ed.) (1969). *The planning of change,* 2nd ed. New York: Holt, Rinehart & Winston.

Bloch, D. (1974). Some crucial terms in nursing: What do they really mean? *Nursing Outlook,* 22, 689-694.

Bruhn, J.G., Cordova, F.D., Williams, J.A., Fuentes, R.G. (1977). The wellness process. *Journal of Community Health,* 2 (3), 209-221.

Bullough, V.L. & Bullough, B. (1971). *The emergence of modern nursing*, 2nd ed. New York: Macmillan.

Bureau, C. (1981). Elaboration et vérification de l'efficacité d'un instrument de collecte d'informations à l'usage des infirmières à domicile. Unpublished master's thesis, Faculty of Nursing, Université de Montréal.

Bureau-Jobin, C. & Pepin, J. (1983). Instrument de collecte de données. In E. Adam, *Etre infirmière*, 2nd ed. (pp. 45-68). Montréal: HRW Ltée.

Bush, H.A. (1979). Models for nursing. *Advances in Nursing Science*, 1 (2), 13-21.

Carpenito, L.J. (1983). *Nursing diagnosis. Application to clinical practice*. New York: Lippincott.

Chinn, P.L. & Jacobs, M.K. (1983). *Theory and nursing: A systematic approach*. St-Louis: Mosby.

Crawford, R. (1977). You are dangerous to your health: The ideology and politics of victim-blaming. *International Journal of Health Services*, 7, 663-680.

Dolan, J. (1978). *Nursing in society: A historical perspective*. Philadelphia: Saunders.

Downs, F.S. (1988). Doctoral education: Our claim to the future. *Nursing Outlook*, 36 (1), 18-20.

Dunn, H.L. (1959). What high-level wellness means. *Canadian Journal of Public Health*, 50, 447-457.

England, M. (1989). Nursing diagnosis: A conceptual framework, In J. Fitzpatrick & A. Whall (Ed.), *Conceptual models of nursing. Analysis and Application*, 2nd ed. (pp. 347-369). Norwalk, CT: Appleton & Lange.

Fawcett, J. (1978). The relationship between theory and research: A double helix. *Advances in Nursing Science*, 1 (1), 49-62.

Fawcett, J. (1985). Theory: Basis for the study and practice of nursing education. *Journal of Nursing Education*, 24, 226-229.

Fawcett, J. (1986). Guest editorial: Conceptual models of nursing, nursing diagnosis, and nursing theory development. *Western Journal of Nursing Research*, 8 (4), 397-399.

Fawcett, J. (1989). *Analysis and evaluation of conceptual models of nursing*, 2nd ed. Philadelphia: F.A. Davis.

Flaskerud, J.H. & Halloran, E.J. (1980). Areas of agreement in nursing theory development. *Advances in Nursing Science*, 3 (1), 1-7.

Ford, L. (1974). The nurse practitioner question (an interview). *American Journal of Nursing*, 74, 2188-2191.

Francis, G. (1967). This thing called problem-solving. *Journal of Nursing Education*, 6 (4), 27-30.

Furukawa, C.Y. & Howe, J.K. (1980). Virginia Henderson. In J.B. George (Ed.), *Nursing Theories. The Base for Professional Nursing Practice*, 2nd ed. The Nursing Theories Conference Group, Englewood Cliffs, NJ: Prentice-Hall.

Gortner, S.R. & Schultz, P.R. (1988). Approaches to nursing science methods. *Image: Journal of Nursing Scholarship*, 20 (1), 22-24.

Greene, J.A. (1979). Science, nursing and nursing science. A conceptual analysis. *Advances in Nursing Science*, 2 (1), 57-64.

Gruending, D.L. (1985). Nursing theory: A vehicle of professionalization? *Journal of Advanced Nursing*, 10, 553-558.

Harmer, B. & Henderson, V. (1955). *Textbook of the principles and practice of nursing*, 5th ed. New York: Macmillan.

Hein, E.C. (1973). *Communication in nursing practice*. Boston: Little, Brown.

Henderson, V. (1964). *The nature of nursing.* American Journal of Nursing, 64 (8), 62-68.

Henderson, V. (1966). *The nature of nursing.* New York: Macmillan.

Henderson, V. (1968). *Basic principles of nursing care*, 4th ed. (brochure). International Council of Nurses.

Henderson, V. & Nite, G. (1978). *Principles and practice of nursing*, 6th ed. New York: Macmillan.

Henderson, V. (1982). The nursing process—is the title right? *Journal of Advanced Nursing*, 7, 103-109.

Henderson, V. (1988). Public address, Montréal.

Jennings, B.M. & Meleis, A.I. (1988). Nursing theory and administrative practice: Agenda for the 1990s. *Advances in Nursing Science*, 10 (3), 56-69.

Jenkins, D.H. (1961). Force field analysis applied to a school situation. In W.G. Bennis, R. Benne, R. Chin (Ed.), *The planning of change* (pp. 238-244). New York: Holt, Rinehart & Winston.

Johnson, D.E. (1974). Development of theory: A requisite for nursing as a primary health profession. *Nursing Research*, 23 (5), 372-377.

Johnson, D.E. (1978). State of the art of theory development in nursing. In *Theory development: What, why, how?* (pp. 1-10). New York: National League for Nursing, no. 15-1708.

Johnson, M.M. (1970). *Problem-solving in nursing practice*. Dubuque, IO: Wm. C. Brown.

Keller, M.J. (1981). Toward a definition of health. *Advances in Nursing Science*, 4 (1), 43-64.

Kim, H.S. (1983). *The nature of theoretical thinking in nursing*. Norwalk, CT: Appleton-Century-Crofts.

Kritek, P.B. (1979). Commentary: The development of nursing diagnosis and theory. *Advances in Nursing Science*, 2 (1), 73-79.

Latourelle, D. (1985). Working with the family and its hospitalized chronically-ill member. In M. Stewart, J. Innes, S. Searl, C. Smillie (Ed.), *Community Health Nursing in Canada* (pp. 348-362). Toronto: Gage Educational Publishing Company.

Levin, R.F., Krainovitch, B.C., Bahrenburg, E. & Mitchell, C.A. (1989). Diagnostic content validity of nursing diagnosis. *Image: Journal of Nursing Scholarship*, 21 (1), 40-44.

Levine, M.E. (1989). The ethics of nursing rhetoric. *Image: Journal of Nursing Scholarship*, 21 (1), 4-6.

Lewin, K. (1961). Quasi-stationary social equilibria and the problem of permanent change. In W.G. Bennis, R. Benne, R. Chin (Ed.), *The planning of change* (pp. 235-238). New York: Holt, Rinehart & Winston.

Maslow, A.H. (1970). *Motivation and personality*, 2nd ed. New York: Harper & Row.

MacQueen, J.S. (1974). A phenomenology of nursing. *Nursing Papers*, 6 (3), 9-19.

Mauksch, H.O. (1966). The organizational context of nursing practice. In F. Davis (Ed.), *The nursing profession: five sociological essays*. New York: John Wiley & Sons.

Meleis, A.I. (1985). *Theoretical nursing. Development and progress*. Philadelphia: Lippincott.

Newman, M. (1986). *Health as expanding consciousness*. St-Louis: Mosby.

Newman, M. (1983). The continuing revolution: A history of nursing science. In N.L. Chaska (Ed.), *The nursing profession. A time to speak* (pp. 385-393). New York: McGraw Hill.

Nadeau, M.A. (1981). *L'évaluation des programmes d'études*. Québec: Université Laval.

Orlando, I.J. (1961). *The dynamic nurse-patient relationship*. New York: G.P. Putnam's Sons.

Parse, R.R. (1987). *Nursing science. Major paradigms, theories and critiques*. Philadelphia: Saunders.

Pepin, J. (1981). Implantation du modèle conceptuel de Virginia Henderson dans un service de soins à domicile. Unpublished master's paper. Faculty of Nursing, Université de Montréal.

Peplau, H.E. (1952). *Interpersonal relations in nursing.* New York: G.P. Putnam's Sons.

Phillips, J.R. (1986). Nursing systems and nursing models. In L.H. Nicoll (Ed.), *Perspectives on nursing theory* (pp. 354-358). Boston: Little, Brown.

Postman, N. & Weingartner, C. (1969). *Teaching as a subversive activity.* New York: Delta.

Riehl, J.P. & Roy, C. (1980). *Conceptual models for nursing practice,* 2nd ed. New York: Appleton-Century-Crofts.

Rogers, C.R. & Stevens, B. (1971). *Person to person.* New York: Pocket Books.

Rogers, C.G. (1973). Conceptual models as guides to clinical nursing specialization. *Journal of Nursing Education,* 12 (4), 2-6.

Rosenbaum, J.N. (1986). Comparison of two theorists on care: Orem and Leininger. *Journal of Advanced Nursing,* 11, 409 419.

Roper, N., Logan, W.W., Tierney, A.J. (1980). *The elements (nursing.* Edinburgh: Churchill Livingstone.

Roy, C. (1984). *Introduction to nursing: An adaptation mode* 2nd ed. Englewood Cliffs, New Jersey: Prentice-Hall.

Roy, C. & Roberts, S.L. (1981). *Theory construction in nursing An adaptation model.* Englewood Cliffs, New Jersey: Prentice-Hall.

Schell, P.L. & Campbell, A.T. (1972). P.O.M.R.—Not just another way to chart. *Nursing Outlook,* 20 (8), 510-514.

Silva, M.C. (1986). Research testing nursing theory: State of the art. *Advances in Nursing Science,* 9 (1), 1-11.

Stainton, M.C., Rankin, J.A. & Calkin, J.D. (1989). The development of a practising nursing faculty. *Journal of Advanced Nursing,* 14, 20-26.

Stevens, B.J. (1979). *Nursing theory. Analysis, application, evaluation.* Boston: Little, Brown.

Travelbee, J. (1966). *Interpersonal aspects of nursing.* Philadelphia: Davis.

Thorndike, E.I. (1940). *Human nature and the social order.* New York: Macmillan.

Ujhely, G. (1968). *Determinants of the nurse-patient relationship.* New York: Springer.

Watson, J. (1979). *Nursing: The philosophy and science of caring.* Boston: Little, Brown.

Watzlawick, P., Beavin, J.H., Jackson, D.D. (1967). *Pragmatics of Human Communication.* New York: Norton.

Woody, M. & Mallison, M. (1974). The problem-oriented system for patient-centered care. *American Journal of Nursing,* 73 (7), 1168-1175.

Woolley, F.R., Warnick, M.W., Kane, R.L., Dyer, E.D. (1974). *Problem-oriented nursing.* New York: Springer.

Wright, L.M. & Leahey, M. (1984). *Nurses and families. A guide to family assessment and intervention.* Philadelphia: Davis.

Wu, R. (1973). *Behavior and illness.* Englewood Cliffs, New Jersey: Prentice-Hall.

Yeo, M. (1989). Integration of nursing theory and nursing ethics. *Advances in Nursing Science,* 11 (3), 33-42.

Yura, H. & Walsh, M.B. (1973). *The nursing process: Assessing, planning, implementing, evaluating,* 2nd ed. New York: Appleton-Century-Crofts.